AF615753

—Diseases and People—

ARTHRITIS

Edward Willett

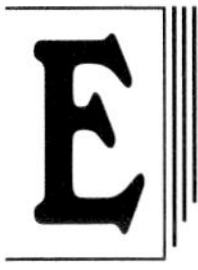

Enslow Publishers, Inc.

40 Industrial Road
Box 398
Berkeley Heights, NJ 07922
USA

PO Box 38
Aldershot
Hants GU12 6BP
UK

http://www.enslow.com

Library of Congress Cataloging-in-Publication Data

Willett, Edward.
Arthritis / Edward Willett
p. cm. — (Diseases and people)
Includes bibliographical references and index.
Summary: Gives a history of the study of arthritis; indicates whom it strikes; and describes symptoms, causes, diagnosis, treatment, prevention, social and economic impact, current research, and future prospects.
ISBN 0-7660-1314-6
1. Arthritis—Juvenile literature. [1. Arthritis. 2. Diseases.] I. Title. II. Series.
RC933 .W545 2000
616.7'22—dc21

99-050696

Printed in the United States of America

10 9 8 7 6 5 4 3 2 1

To Our Readers:
All Internet addresses in this book were active and appropriate when we went to press. Any comments or suggestions can be sent by e-mail to Comments@enslow.com or to the address on the back cover.

Illustration Credits: The Arthritis Foundation, pp. 8, 11, 13, 35, 37, 39, 58, 59, 67, 79; © Corel Corporation, p. 30; courtesy of Bayer Aspirin, pp. 22, 61; courtesy of the Sharper Image, pp. 70, 81 (bottom); DíAMAR Interactive Corp., p. 89; Edward Willett, p. 75; Enslow Publishers, Inc., p. 6, 81 (top), 82, 92; Kathiann M. Kowalski, p. 71; National Cancer Institute, p. 50; National Institutes of Health, pp. 45, 63; National Library of Medicine, p. 20.

Cover Illustration: The Arthritis Foundation.

Contents

PROFILE

ARTHRITIS

What is it? The term *arthritis* refers to more than one hundred different conditions that cause pain, swelling, and limited movement in the body's joints and other tissues that connect bones.

Who gets it? All ages, all races, both sexes. Although the most common form of arthritis, osteoarthritis, is found mainly in older people, the most severe form, rheumatoid arthritis, can strike children and young adults.

How do you get it? There are almost as many causes of arthritis as there are types. Rheumatoid arthritis results from a disturbance in the body's immune system that causes it to attack its own tissues. Osteoarthritis is a breakdown of the protective cushion of cartilage covering the ends of bones where they meet to form a joint, and can be caused simply by the wear and tear of aging. Bacterial infections also cause some types of arthritis.

What are the symptoms? Swelling in one or more joints; stiffness, especially in the early morning, for more than a few minutes; recurring pain or tenderness in a joint; restricted movement in a joint; obvious redness or warmth in a joint; or unexplained weight loss, fever, or weakness, combined with joint pain.

How is it treated? The relatively few cases of arthritis caused by bacterial infection can be treated with antibiotics. For most types of arthritis, however, there is no cure, so treatment focuses on easing the symptoms. The goal is to reduce pain and swelling so the patient can carry on a normal life. Most forms of arthritis are treated with general anti-inflammatory drugs such as aspirin, ibuprofen, and cortisone.

How can it be prevented? There is no known way of preventing rheumatoid arthritis. However, the risk of developing osteoarthritis can be reduced by controlling weight, avoiding joint injuries from overuse or accidents, and exercising regularly. Even people already suffering from arthritis can prevent some of its worst effects with regular exercise, which keeps joints and muscles as strong and limber as possible.

RESERVED
PARKING
PENALTY
$100 1st OFFENSE
SUBSEQUENT OFFENSES
$100 MIN AND/OR
UP TO 90 DAYS
COMMUNITY SERVICE
TOW-AWAY ZONE

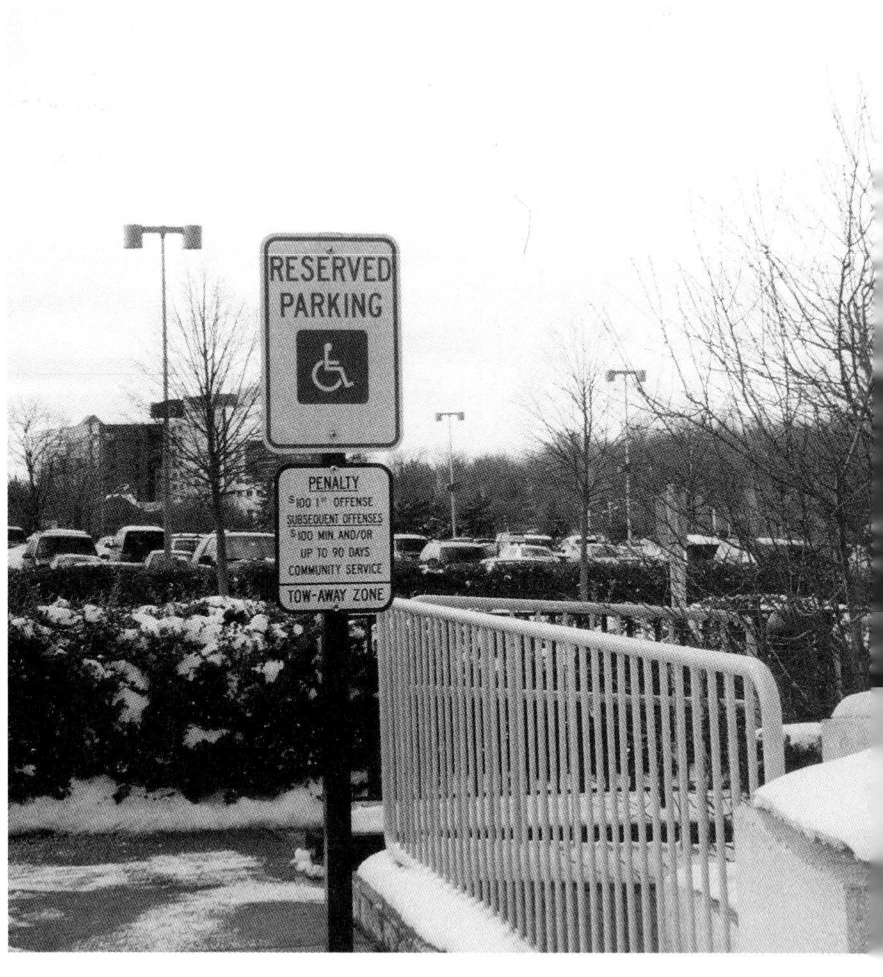

The passage of the Americans with Disabilities Act in 1990, among other provisions, set aside easily accessible parking spaces, which are helpful to persons with severe arthritis.

1

Oh, My Aching Joints!

Becky was an active four-year-old who was normally full of cheerful chatter. Over a period of time, however, a teacher at her childcare center noticed changes in Becky's behavior. Sometimes she sat all by herself in the playground instead of running around with the other children. She became irritable. Finally, she started to avoid putting weight on her left leg, even though her teacher could see nothing wrong with it.

The teacher reported her observations to Becky's parents, who then asked their daughter if she hurt anywhere. Becky said she did not, but over the next few weeks she began limping, and her knee became swollen and hot. Soon she began waking up in the morning crying, admitting that she hurt.

Becky's parents took her to her doctor, who examined her knee, then ordered some laboratory tests. The results indicated that the doctor's first suspicion was correct: Becky had juvenile rheumatoid arthritis.

Becky's parents were very upset. They thought arthritis only happened to older people. They wondered if it was somehow their fault. Could Becky have caught the disease at the childcare center?

The doctor told Becky's parents not to blame themselves. He reassured them that the disease is not contagious. He also told them that most children with arthritis improve, and do not suffer any long-term joint damage or disabilities, but he also warned them that the disease is different in every child.

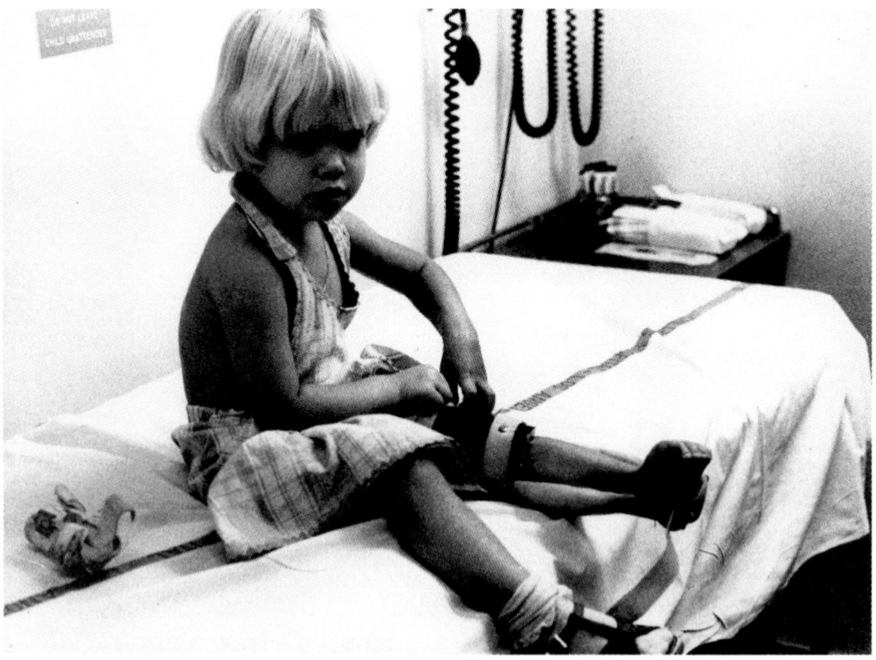

Arthritis can strike even very young children. Fortunately, most juvenile arthritis patients grow out of their disease and suffer no lasting effects.

That meant he could not tell them how long Becky would suffer from arthritis or how severe it would be. All the doctors could do, he said, was see that Becky got the necessary medication, physical therapy, and exercise, to try to control her symptoms and keep her as active as possible.[1]

✦ ✦ ✦

Sarah had suffered from occasional back pain for years, but she still lived a very active life. However, during the year she turned seventy-two, her knees started to hurt, too, and the back pain grew so bad she had to cut the time she spent on some of her favorite activities, like golf. Her hands began to change, too, her knuckles becoming so enlarged that she had trouble getting her wedding ring on and off her finger. It even became difficult for her to grip some ordinary objects, such as jar lids.

Sarah found it particularly hard to get around in the morning. She discovered that if she sat still for a long time, at a church service, for instance, her joints would "freeze up" on her, making it difficult for her to move quickly or smoothly.

Sarah went to her doctor, who diagnosed her condition as osteoarthritis. The doctor prescribed aspirin to relieve her pain and to reduce the swelling in the joints, and a regular program of exercise. Now Sarah is once again golfing regularly and swimming laps several times a week, although occasionally she has days when she hurts so much she has to walk with a cane. Still, Sarah says, "Osteoarthritis can be annoying, and it's hard to keep a good attitude when the pain is bad. But I've learned to live with it. If you don't keep moving, you're a goner."[2]

More Than One Hundred Kinds

Becky's and Sarah's diseases are very different, but they are both forms of arthritis. In all, there are more than one hundred kinds.

The word arthritis comes from two Greek words, *arthron*, which means joint, and *itis*, which means inflammation. Inflammation, the body's natural response to injury, causes swelling, redness, warmth, and pain; so arthritis, literally, means "painful, swollen joints." Many different conditions can cause the joints to become painful and swollen; therefore there are many different types of arthritis.

As if that were not confusing enough, some forms of arthritis do not cause inflammation in the joints at all! Instead, they affect other types of tissues, including muscle and the connective tissues that make up or support the body's structures: tendons, cartilage, blood vessels, and internal organs.

All the various forms of arthritis are also often called "rheumatic diseases."[3]

Taken together, rheumatic diseases affect nearly 43 million Americans—or one out of every six. That makes arthritis one of the most common health problems in the United States. Nearly 3 million Americans suffer so severely from the effects of arthritis that they have trouble with everyday activities such as walking, dressing, or bathing.[4]

Three Women for Every Two Men

Most forms of arthritis strike more women than men; scientists do not know why. More than 75 percent of rheumatoid arthritis patients, for example, are women.[5] Osteoarthritis, on the other hand, strikes both men and women, but it tends to show up in women earlier than in men.[6] The Centers for Disease Control and Prevention in Atlanta, Georgia, reports that for every two men with some form of arthritis, there are three women. In fact, arthritis is the most frequent health problem for women. It is nearly three times as common as the second-most frequent health problem, high blood pressure, which affects 8 million women.[7]

Prevalence of Arthritis by Age

Age	No. in the thousands	% of Group
≤ 16	285	0.5
17–25	873	2.9
25–34	2,862	6.6
35–44	4,778	12.7
45–54	5,757	22.6
55–64	7,699	36.5
65–74	8,273	45.4
75–84	5,501	55.2
85+	1,714	57.1

This chart from the Arthritis Foundation shows the numbers and percentages of people in the United States who get arthritis, according to their ages.

The one exception to the pattern of more women being affected than men is the form of arthritis known as gout. It tends to strike more men than women and at a younger age. Gout, which affects as many as eight hundred forty out of every one hundred thousand people, is strongly associated with obesity, high blood pressure, and diabetes.[8] Having gout simply adds to the problems of people who are already suffering from these other medical difficulties.

Some forms of arthritis can even shorten people's lives. For instance, patients with rheumatoid arthritis do not generally live quite as long as people who do not have the disease. Similarly, the form called lupus and another form of arthritis called scleroderma, both of which can damage other organs besides the joints, can shorten a person's life span.

Even the medical treatments for arthritis can sometimes be fatal. Every year, one hundred seven thousand Americans are sent to the hospital and sixteen thousand five hundred die from the side effects of nonsteroidal anti-inflammatory drugs (NSAIDs), the most common treatment for arthritis.[9] NSAIDs can cause serious bleeding in the stomach.

Not Just Old People

Becky's parents were not alone in believing that arthritis is a condition that primarily affects older people. Many people do not realize that arthritis can strike anyone. In fact, "Arthritis can strike people of all ages, not just someone's grandmother or great aunt," says Dr. Robert P. Kimberly, director of the Multipurpose Arthritis and Musculoskeletal Disease Center, and professor of medicine at Cornell University Medical College in New York City.[10]

Still, the most common form of arthritis is osteoarthritis, which affects nearly 16 million Americans. It is one of the leading causes of disability in adults over age sixty-five.[11] That is because osteoarthritis is probably caused by the natural, regular wear and tear on our joints over the course of our lives. As a result, the longer we live, the more likely we are to develop osteoarthritis.

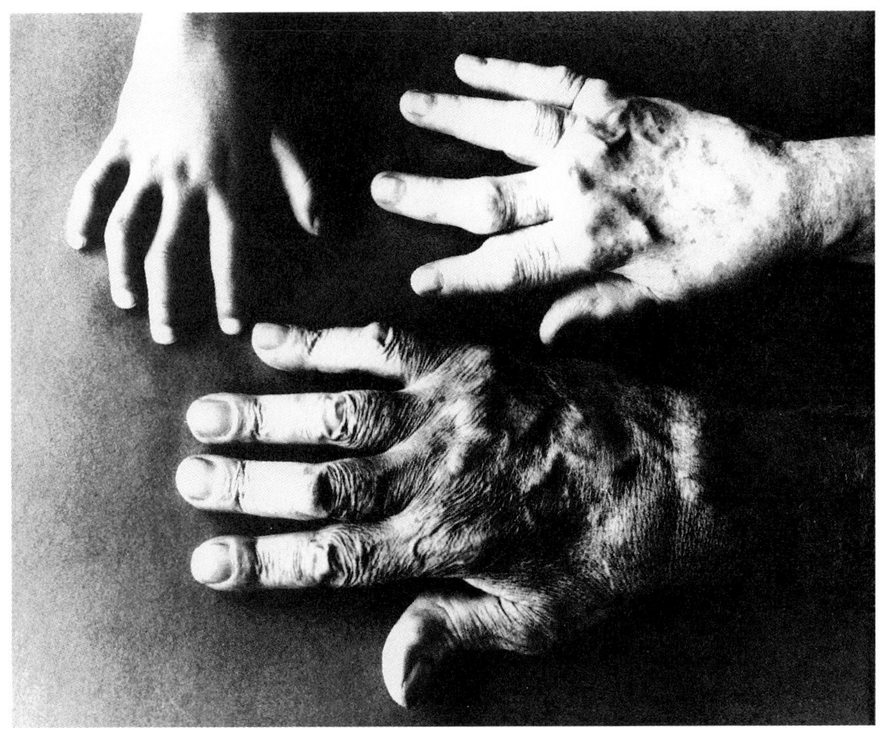

Many people believe arthritis affects only older people. They do not realize that the disease can strike people of any race or age.

Normally, the ends of our bones are cushioned by pieces of smooth, stringy tissue called cartilage. If this cartilage deteriorates, due to age or injury, the bones at the ends of joints get thicker. In addition, extra bony growths, called osteophytes, or bone spurs, may form. Any or all of these changes can mean that the joint does not work as smoothly as it used to. It may also become stiff and painful.

Whereas osteoarthritis affects men and women in more or less even proportions, it rarely shows up until people are in their forties or fifties, and it generally strikes women earlier than men. On the other hand, the most severe form of arthritis, rheumatoid arthritis, is quite different, and can attack people of any age, although its most common victims are women in their forties.[12]

Osteoarthritis results from damage to joints, but rheumatoid arthritis affects previously undamaged joints. No one knows what triggers rheumatoid arthritis. It seems to be caused by a malfunction in the immune system, which normally defends the body against infection and helps the body repair itself. In rheumatoid arthritis, the immune system starts attacking the body instead of defending it.

It is estimated that approximately one percent of the population of the United States, or roughly 2.5 million people, have rheumatoid arthritis.[13] There are many other forms of arthritis, with many different causes. For example, gout is caused by a buildup in the body of a body chemical called uric acid, and psoriatic arthritis results from a complication of psoriasis, a common skin disease.

An Expensive Disease

Because it affects so many people, arthritis has a huge impact on society, costing the United States economy alone $65 billion per year in medical care and lost wages.[14] That cost, and the number of people suffering from some form of arthritis, will climb as the baby boomers—the large group of people born from the late 1940s to the mid-1960s—get older. By 2020, about 60 million Americans will have arthritis.[15]

On an individual basis, arthritis sufferers have to deal not only with daily pain, but also with the uncertain course of their disease. Many types of arthritis have an on-again, off-again pattern, which means the physical effects can change from day to day and even from hour to hour. In extreme cases, arthritis can severely handicap movement, or even confine people to a wheelchair.

Because arthritis is so common, even those who may never suffer from the disease themselves almost certainly have a friend or family member who does.

For all of these reasons, it is important to understand what arthritis is, what its symptoms are, how it can be treated, and how some types can be prevented.

2

A History of Arthritis

Between three thousand and five thousand years ago, a community of humans lived in what is now the northwestern part of the state of Alabama. We know very little about these people, because the only traces of them that remain are some bones dug up from the shores of the Tennessee River in the 1930s.

However, in 1988, anthropologist Kenneth R. Turner of the University of Alabama in Tuscaloosa learned one important fact about six of these ancient humans, something they had in common with many people alive today: They suffered from rheumatoid arthritis.

Turner and his colleagues noticed bone loss of these specimens near their hand, arm, leg, and foot joints, which is typical of rheumatoid arthritis damage. X rays of the joints showed damage nearly identical to that which shows up on the X rays of modern-day sufferers.[1]

Those six ancient Alabamans are the earliest known sufferers of rheumatoid arthritis among modern humans. They are not the earliest known human victims of arthritis, however; that "honor" belongs to some Neanderthal people whose bones were excavated in Germany in 1855. Those bones, from one hundred fifty thousand years ago, showed evidence of osteoarthritis.[2]

Since that time, millions more people have suffered from all the various types of arthritis.

It's All Greek

Certainly the ancient Greeks knew about arthritis, since they gave us the word to describe the condition. It was a Greek, Aurelius Cornelius Celsus, who lived in Rome at the time of Christ, who gave us the first written description of inflammation: swelling, redness, heat, and pain.[3]

Although they recognized the symptoms of inflammation, the Greeks didn't understand what caused it. They believed all disease was caused by an imbalance of fluids they called "humors." If a knee became sore and swollen, they thought it was because excess humors had flowed into that joint.

Another word for arthritis, *rheumatism,* was also created by an ancient Greek, probably a physician named Galen who worked in Rome in the second century A.D.[4] The Greek word *reuma* means stream or flow, so *rheumatism* means the flow of humors.

The Romans were familiar with arthritis, as well. Some historians estimate that more than 70 percent of Romans over the age of thirty were afflicted with some form of arthritis. Historians speculate that one of the main functions of the famous Roman baths was to help ease the population's aching joints.[5] The Roman emperor Diocletian even exempted citizens with severe arthritis from paying taxes. Perhaps he felt that simply having arthritis was taxing enough for his citizens.

The Greek belief in humors carried on for many centuries. The form of arthritis called gout gets its name from the Latin word *gutta*, which means drop. In the thirteenth century, people referred to all forms of arthritis as gout, and believed it occurred because humors flowed into the inflamed joints, drop by drop.[6]

Non-European cultures were also familiar with arthritis, an indication of just how widespread the disease has always been. For example, as far back as 123 A.D., there is a reference to a condition that certainly sounds like arthritis in an East Indian story called *Caraka Samhita.* It describes a disease where swollen, painful joints initially strike the hands and feet, then spread to other parts of the body, causing loss of appetite, and occasionally fever.[7]

A true scientific discussion of arthritis was not written for a few more centuries. One of the first books on arthritis was written in 1591 by Guillaume de Baillou (1538–1616), a French physician and dean of the University of Paris medical faculty. He described the suffering of those with the condition he called *rheumatisme*:

> The whole body hurts, in some the face is flushed; pain is most severe around the joints, so that the slightest movement of the foot, hand or finger causes a cry of pain. . . . At night . . . the pain becomes more serious and the patient cannot sleep.[8]

About eighty years later, in 1676, the English physician Thomas Sydenham wrote about a long-term, chronic disease that affects many joints and can cause deformed fingers—probably rheumatoid arthritis. Sydenham was also the first person to differentiate gout from other forms of arthritis.[9]

By the eighteenth century, gout as we know it today had become associated with high living, superior social status, and longevity. Many prominent men suffered from gout, from kings and statesmen like Thomas Jefferson to artists and inventors like Benjamin Franklin, probably because the upper-class diet of the time was rich in meats, fat, and alcohol, and low in vegetables and carbohydrates. This diet can contribute to the development of gout.

During the eighteenth century the idea that gout was somehow associated with longevity mistakenly arose because, at the time, the average life expectancy was only around thirty years. Since gout is more prevalent in people over the age of forty-five, it seemed as though gout and longevity went hand in hand.

Benjamin Franklin and Thomas Jefferson were not the only well-known men affected by gout during the American Revolution. British statesman William Pitt the Elder, first earl of Chatham, suffered an attack of gout that kept him from attending Parliament, the British government assembly, where

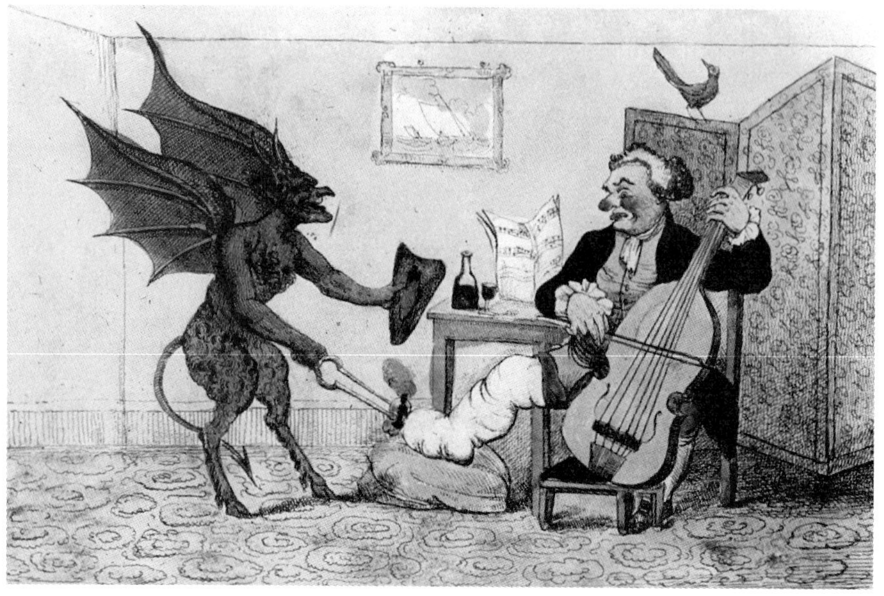

This etching made in 1815 entitled "The Origin of Gout" illustrates how painful gout can be—in this case as painful as a demon applying hot coals to a person's toe.

he most likely would have stopped the passage of a tax on tea. That tax led to the Boston Tea Party—and eventually to independence for England's American colonies.[10]

Searching for a Treatment

Scientists still had no idea what caused arthritis, but they were already looking for better ways to treat it. In ancient times, the Greek physician Hippocrates had recommended that women suffering pain in childbirth should chew on bark from the willow tree. In 1763, an English clergyman named Edmund Stone noted that remedies made from willow bark could also help reduce rheumatic fever and pain.[11] We now know that willow bark contains a chemical called salicylate—the active ingredient in aspirin (see page 23), still one of the basic drugs prescribed to reduce pain and inflammation.

Rheumatoid arthritis was not officially recognized and described until 1800, in a thesis published by Austin-Jacob Landré-Beauvais of Paris. It was not called rheumatoid arthritis until 1859, when Sir Alfred Garrod, a physician in London, proposed that name, although he intended it to apply to a large variety of joint problems, not just the distinct disease we call rheumatoid arthritis today.[12] It was also in the early nineteenth century, in a book by Sir Charles Scudmore, that the first reference appeared about the idea that arthritis may run in families.[13]

During the nineteenth century scientific research began to be conducted into the causes of arthritis. Scientists had just begun to realize that many diseases were caused by bacteria, thanks primarily to Robert Koch's discovery in 1875 of the organism that causes anthrax, a serious disease of livestock. In the early 1890s, a researcher in Paris named M. Bouchard studied arthritic joints, taking samples from them to try to discover what type of bacteria had caused them to become inflamed. Although the paper Bouchard published in 1894 was widely quoted, we now know that Bouchard's samples must have been contaminated, since the bacteria he mentioned in the report do not cause arthritis.

At the beginning of the twentieth century new theories about the causes of arthritis were put forward. Some scientists

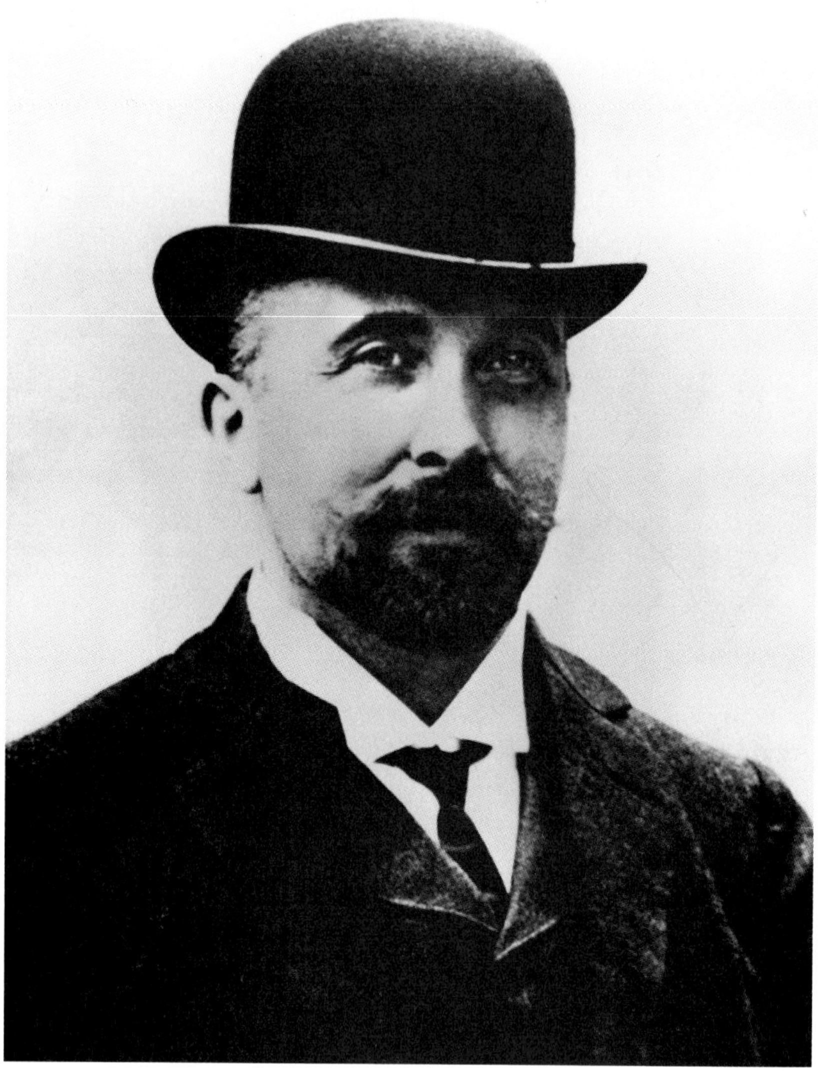

Felix Hoffmann, a chemist working for the German drug company called Bayer, discovered a stable form of acetylsalicylic acid (ASA), the active ingredient in aspirin. Hoffmann discovered ASA in his search for a more effective, safe treatment for his father, who was crippled by arthritis.

The Development of Aspirin[14]

Aspirin is such a common drug that we take it for granted, but we really should not.

The active ingredient in willow bark, salicylate, was isolated in 1838 by Raffaelle Piria, a young Italian chemist working at the Sorbonne University in Paris. At the time, salicylate was used not only to relieve pain, but also in the making of the dyes used to color cloth. Its use increased even more in 1860 after German chemist Hermann Kolgbe figured out a way to manufacture it out of phenol, a chemical derived from coal tar.

Salicylate had serious side effects. It was very hard on the stomach, for one thing, and it tasted so awful that it made some patients sick. In 1897 Felix Hoffmann, a chemist working for the German drug company Bayer, came up with a less harmful form of salicylic acid: acetylsalicylic acid, or ASA for short. Hoffmann had a personal reason for finding a less harsh version of the drug: His father suffered from arthritis, and couldn't tolerate salicylate.

A chemist in Strasbourg, France, named Charles Frederic Gerhardt, had synthesized ASA four decades earlier (although it wasn't chemically pure enough to be used as a drug), so Bayer couldn't patent the substance in most countries. What the company could do, however, was come up with a trademark name for it. Bayer chose the name "aspirin."

ASA has been marketed under many other brand names since then—Anacin, for example—but Bayer got there first, and today "aspirin," rather than the tongue-twisting "acetylsalicylic acid" is the generic term for the first of the class of medicines that are today called nonsteroidal anti-inflammatory drugs (NSAIDs).

thought the inflammation of a joint must be due to poisons released by bacteria elsewhere in the body. As a result, many people underwent operations in which infected teeth, tonsils, and even major organs were removed, the theory being that the infected parts were causing the arthritis.

Although these operations were both unnecessary and dangerous, there was a kernel of truth in the idea that bacteria could cause arthritis. Indeed, several types of bacterial infections can result in inflammation of the joints.

Viruses, too, can cause some forms of arthritis. Bacteria are tiny, but they are complete living organisms. Like other living organisms, they eat, excrete, and reproduce. Viruses are even smaller than bacteria, but they are not complete organisms. As Martinus Beijerinck, an Amsterdam microbiologist, realized in 1897, viruses can only reproduce by taking over a living cell and changing it, so that the cell produces more viruses, instead of doing its intended work.[15] Since Beijerinck's time, researchers have discovered many viruses that can cause arthritis, including the viruses that cause rubella (German measles), hepatitis, mumps, and AIDS.[16]

However, so far neither bacteria nor viruses have been found to be the cause of osteoarthritis or rheumatoid arthritis, the most common forms of the condition.

Recognizing Different Forms

Osteoarthritis was named by John Kent Spender, a physician in Bath, England, in 1888. However, doctors did not realize osteoarthritis was different from rheumatoid arthritis until early in the twentieth century, after they had examined the joint damage caused by both diseases under the microscope.[17] *Osteo* means "bone," and was included in the name in reference to the changes in the joint bones caused by the loss of padding between them.

With the recognition that osteoarthritis and rheumatoid arthritis were different and distinct came a number of theories as to what caused rheumatoid arthritis. The modern notion that it is a disease in which the immune system attacks the body was first put forward by Sir McFarlane Burnet, head of the Research Institute of Melbourne, Australia, in 1930.[18]

Widespread research into all kinds of arthritis has occurred in just the last few decades, and many new treatments have been developed. One pioneer in the study and treatment of rheumatoid arthritis was Philip Showalter Hench, an American pathologist who, during the 1930s, noticed that patients suffering from rheumatoid arthritis often improved when they were stricken by jaundice. Jaundice is a condition that occurs when the blood contains too much bilirubin, a substance produced by the liver. Hench also noticed that pregnant women suffered less from their arthritis than other arthritis sufferers. He reasoned that if he could find a substance in the blood common to both jaundice and pregnancy, it might lead him to a new treatment for rheumatoid arthritis.

His research eventually led him to the adrenal glands, part of the endocrine system, which produce several hormones. One of these, cortisol, is released in increased amounts in a person with jaundice, and during pregnancy and other times of stress or injury, and can produce a feeling of well-being, or even exhilaration. Hench's colleague Edward Kendell managed to produce a synthetic version of cortisol, which Hench called cortisone. In tests carried out at the Mayo Clinic in Rochester, Minnesota, in 1948, cortisone injections enabled patients who had been almost crippled to regain the use of their joints. Another hormone, adrenocorticopic hormone (ACTH), produced by the pituitary gland, also worked well. ACTH stimulates the adrenal glands to produce cortisol.

Although synthetic adrenal hormones, collectively called corticosteroids, have since been proven to have dangerous side effects, Hench and Kendell's experiments opened up an important new field of study for the treatment of rheumatoid arthritis. Even more importantly, corticosteroids transformed systemic lupus erythematosus (lupus, for short), a disease in which the body's immune system attacks the body's own tissue, from a disease that was almost always fatal into one that is chronic, or incurable, but manageable. (Because one of the symptoms of lupus can be joint inflammation, lupus is considered a form of arthritis.) Hench and Kendell shared the 1950 Nobel Prize for physiology in the category of medicine for their work.[19]

In 1948, when Hench and Kendell began testing corticosteroids, another important discovery was made. Scientists found that a natural antibody called the "rheumatoid factor" appears in the blood of people suffering from arthritis. A test for that antibody was developed, and is now one of the standard blood tests performed to help diagnose rheumatoid arthritis.[20]

The Last Fifty Years

In the fifty years since Hench and Kendall's experiments, enormous strides have been made in the field of arthritis research. We have learned to classify, diagnose, and manage many types of arthritis. Chronic gout, for instance, was once a serious disease: Now it can be controlled by medication. Lupus used to kill many more people than it does now. Arthritis caused by rheumatic fever has almost been wiped out in the United States.

One great stride has been the increasing use of surgery to treat arthritis. The first total hip replacement surgery was carried out in England in 1938. Today, artificial hips, knees, and other joints help people regain movement that once would have been lost forever.

Research continues in many different fields, including immunology (the study of how the body protects itself from disease), genetics (the study of how characteristics are passed from generation to generation), and microbiology (the study of microorganisms, including the bacteria and viruses that cause disease). Scientists want to know what makes joints become inflamed and why some people are more likely to suffer from arthritis than others. Other researchers want to know what causes the cartilage and bone to deteriorate and bring on osteoarthritis. Better understanding should lead to new and better treatments in the years to come.

In addition, there is much better support available today for people with arthritis than there once was. One important organization that contributed to the fight against arthritis, and the fight to improve life for people with arthritis, is the Arthritis Foundation.

Its origins go back to 1948, when there were only seven locations in the country where physicians and medical students could learn about arthritis, and only six treatment and research centers. The American Rheumatism Association (ARA), made up of approximately three hundred physicians with advanced knowledge and training in rheumatic diseases, felt this situation was unacceptable. Inspired by the successes of the medical community in treating such conditions as polio, the ARA played an important role in forming the Arthritis and Rheumatism Foundation (today shortened to the Arthritis Foundation). In addition to providing information and support for people suffering from arthritis, the foundation has provided more than $200 million to more than seventeen hundred physicians and scientists for research.[21]

Greater public attention to arthritis in the United States was also demonstrated by the National Arthritis Act. Signed into law on January 4, 1975, the act authorized substantial expansion of resources for arthritis research, training, public education, and treatment. It recommended the establishment of comprehensive arthritis centers, an institute of arthritis in the National Institutes of Health (NIH), an arthritis data bank, and development of a long-range plan to address the various problems of arthritis across the nation.

The first three of the act's major recommendations have been realized. The Arthritis Foundation recently released the *National Arthritis Action Plan: A Public Health Strategy* to meet the final recommendation. The goal of the plan is to make everyone more aware of the impact of arthritis, what can be done to prevent or delay it, and what can be done to improve the quality of life of people with arthritis.[22]

Arthritis vs. Artists and Athletes

Over the centuries, many people have suffered from arthritis. One of the most famous sufferers was the French impressionist Pierre-Auguste Renoir, recognized as one of the greatest painters of the late nineteenth century. Today Renoir's paintings hang in great museums like the Louvre in Paris and the Metropolitan Museum of Art in New York City.

Renoir, who was born in Limoges, France, in 1841, lived until 1919, but his best known paintings all date from the nineteenth century. That is partly because, for the last twenty years of his life, Renoir's hands were severely crippled by arthritis. Nevertheless, he continued to paint, using a brush strapped to his arm.[23]

In the twentieth century, some of the most famous sufferers of arthritis have been professional athletes. Harry Heilmann, who led the American League in batting four times while he was with the Detroit Tigers during the 1920s, and who holds the second all-time best batting average record of .342, was forced to sit out the entire 1931 baseball season because of arthritis in his wrists. His career ended early in 1932, when he retired after just fifteen games.[24]

Baseball legend Mickey Mantle, who scored 536 home runs with the New York Yankees during the 1950s and 1960s,

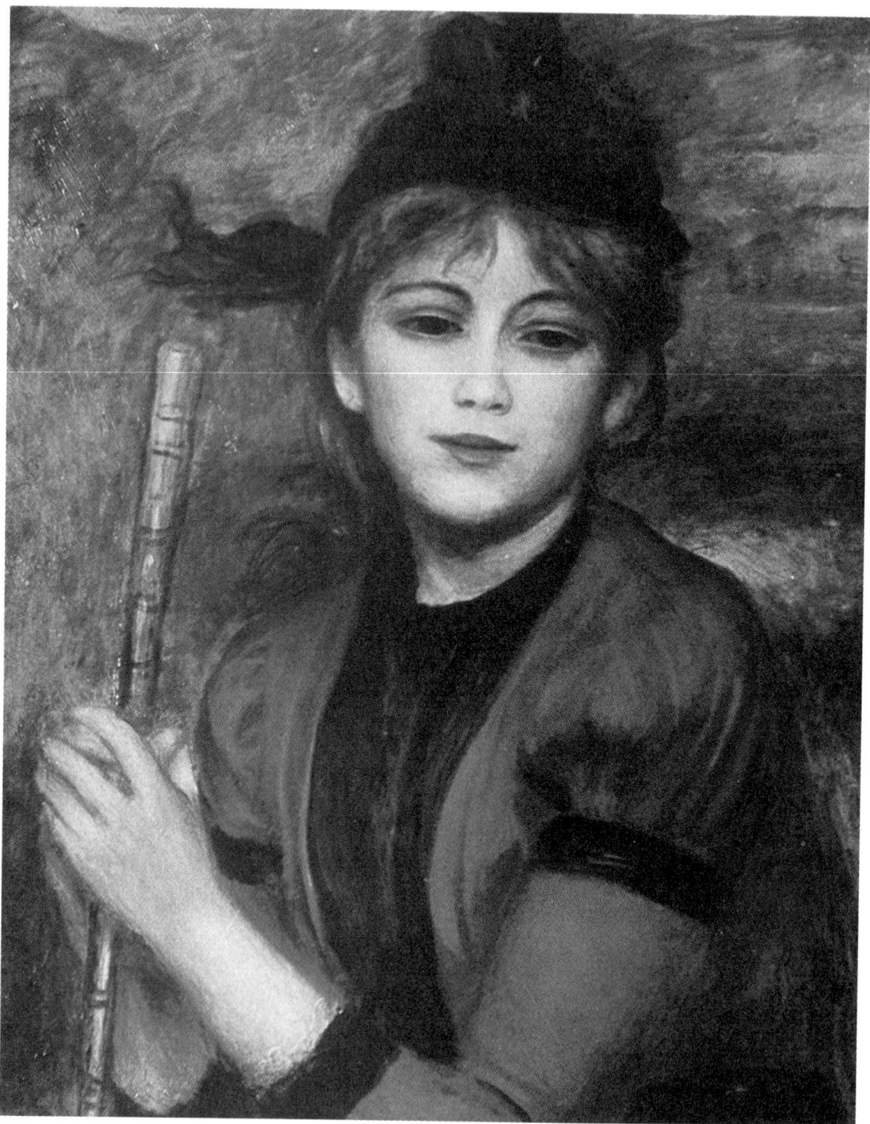

For the last twenty years of his life, French impressionist painter Pierre-Auguste Renoir was crippled with rhematoid arthritis. Although he could no longer walk and his fingers were stiff, he continued to paint by strapping a paintbrush onto his arm. This portrait by Renoir is called "The Excursionist."

was forced to retire from baseball when he was only thirty-six years old because of recurring injuries to his knees. Years later, he was diagnosed with osteoarthritis, probably the result of those injuries.[25]

Still more recently, Britt Burns, a left-handed pitcher who won seventy games for the Chicago White Sox from 1980 through 1985, was forced out of baseball at the age of twenty-six. Osteoarthritis in his right hip became so severe that Burns could hardly put on his right shoe without help.[26]

Many famous performers have also suffered from arthritis. Lucille Ball, one of the most famous comedians of the twentieth century, was diagnosed with rheumatoid arthritis at the age of seventeen. At the time, she was living in New York, struggling through theater school and working as a chorus girl and model. One day while being fitted for a modeling session, after several days of pneumonia and fever, Ball felt terrible pains in both her legs, as if they were on fire. A doctor told her the pains were symptoms of arthritis.

Treatment was unsuccessful, and Ball had to return to her parents' home in Jamestown, New York, where she was all but bedridden. When the pain finally subsided and she was able to stand again, her left leg was shorter than her right leg, and it pulled sideways. She had to wear a twenty-pound weight in one of her black orthopedic shoes to try to correct the problem. Although Ball continued to suffer from residual pains, she soon recovered enough to take a part offered her by the Jamestown Players, and eventually she went on to make a name for herself as the "queen of comedy," especially of vigorous physical comedy.[27]

Another celebrity who has battled arthritis is actor James Coburn. In 1990, Coburn suffered so badly from rheumatoid arthritis that he could barely walk.[28] Ironically, in 1999, he won the Academy Award for best supporting actor for his role in a movie called *Affliction.*

As Coburn and Ball illustrate, it is possible to manage arthritis successfully and continue to have a full, productive life and career.

3

What Is Arthritis?

Over a period of time, Mary, a forty-two-year-old secretary with two school-age children, began to notice a nagging discomfort in her joints. At first it was just her wrists and fingers that hurt; then it was her knees. Her joints felt the worst in the morning; if she took a hot shower, she usually felt better.

The pain came and went. Sometimes she felt achy all over. As time went on, however, the pains became more constant. Mary's fingers became swollen, and she felt so stiff in the morning it was hard to get out of bed. The stiffness would wear off in a couple of hours, but Mary decided it was time to talk to her doctor.

Her family physician referred her to an arthritis specialist, called a rheumatologist, who examined her thoroughly and conducted several tests. Afterward, he told Mary that she had rheumatoid arthritis. He began to explain to her how, exactly, arthritis affects the joints.

How a Joint Works

A joint is a place where two bones come together. There are many different types of joints. Some, like the joints where the various bones in the skull come together, are fixed, so they cannot move. Some, like the joints in the spine where the vertebrae meet, allow a small amount of movement. Others, the ones we usually think of when we think of joints—hips, knees, elbows, and knuckles, for example—allow a much greater range of movement. Altogether, there are more than two hundred bones in the human skeleton, connected by nearly one hundred fifty joints.[1]

The connecting ends of the bones in the joints that allow for motion are covered in cartilage. This smooth, tough, and spongy material works like a shock absorber and also allows the joint to move easily. To get an idea of how flexible and strong cartilage is, bend your ears. They're made of cartilage covered with skin.

Surrounding the joint is a strong capsule formed by thick, cord-like fibers called ligaments, which are anchored to the bone on either side of the joint. The ligaments help keep the bones lined up properly.

The joint capsule is lined with the thin, velvety synovial membrane. This membrane, which is crisscrossed with blood vessels and nerve endings, produces a thick, clear liquid called the synovial fluid. This fluid acts like the grease on a bicycle chain, lubricating the joint and helping it to move easily. The synovial fluid also nourishes the cartilage and removes any waste products, such as dead cells.[2]

A similar lubricating liquid is produced by small fluid-filled sacs outside the joint called bursae. Joints are moved by muscles, special tissues that can contract and relax. The muscles are attached to the bone by tendons, strong bands similar to ligaments. The fluid from the bursae helps muscles, tendons, and bones slide smoothly over one another.

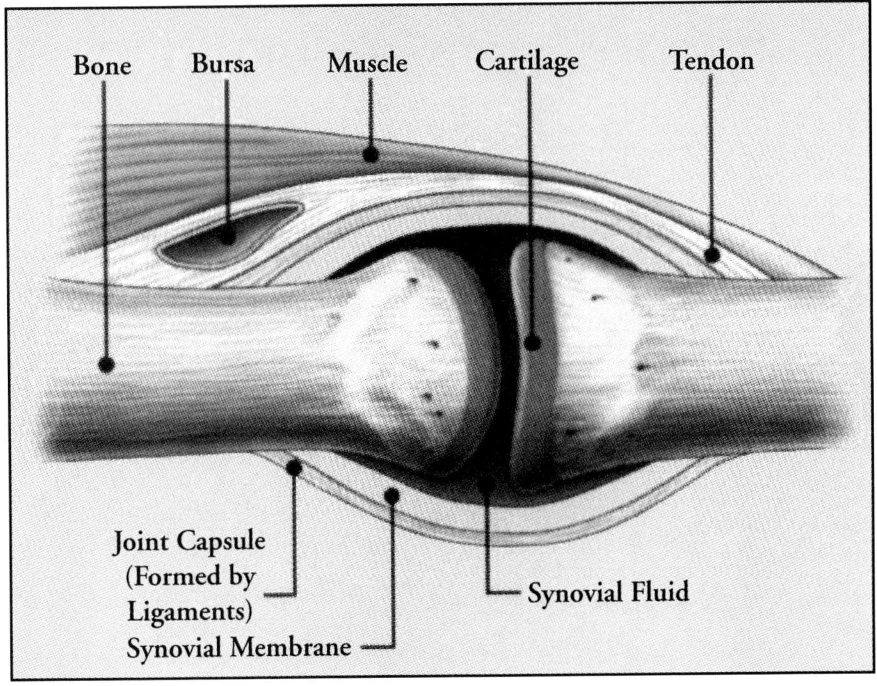

This diagram shows the parts of a normal joint capsule.

When a person has arthritis, something goes wrong, and the parts of the joint no longer move smoothly. What effect that has on the person's life depends on which joint is affected.

People whose hands are afflicted with arthritis, for instance, may have trouble buttoning buttons, typing, holding a pen, opening doors, brushing their teeth, or even feeding themselves (because they find it hard to grip a spoon or fork). A person whose knees are affected has difficulty walking, climbing stairs, sitting down (and standing up again), taking a bath, or getting out of bed in the morning. Arthritic hips also make it hard to walk, sit, or stand for long periods. Arthritis in the neck can make it painful to turn your head. Arthritis in the back makes it difficult to bend over, pick things up, lift heavy objects, or even sleep well.

Usually, our joints are parts of the body we tend to take for granted, right up until the moment when they don't work well any longer.

Osteoarthritis

The most common form of arthritis is osteoarthritis. *Osteo* means bone, but osteoarthritis actually has more to do with the tissue between the bones than the bones themselves. Sometimes called "joint failure" or the "wear and tear disease," osteoarthritis is the result of the degeneration of tissue and the growth of bony spurs (osteophytes) in a joint. This combination of conditions causes stiffness, pain, and sometimes swelling.[3]

Osteoarthritis begins with changes in the joint cartilage. It becomes soft and pitted. That, in turn, means it loses its elasticity and strength. As the cartilage thins, the bone ends begin to rub together, causing pain in the joint.

Since the lengths of the ligaments don't change as the cartilage thins, eventually they become too long for the joint. This means they are no longer holding the bones of the joint together as tightly, which can make the joint unstable.[4]

The bones that are rubbing together respond to the damage being caused by growing out at the sides, becoming more dense, and developing bony spurs where the ligaments attach.

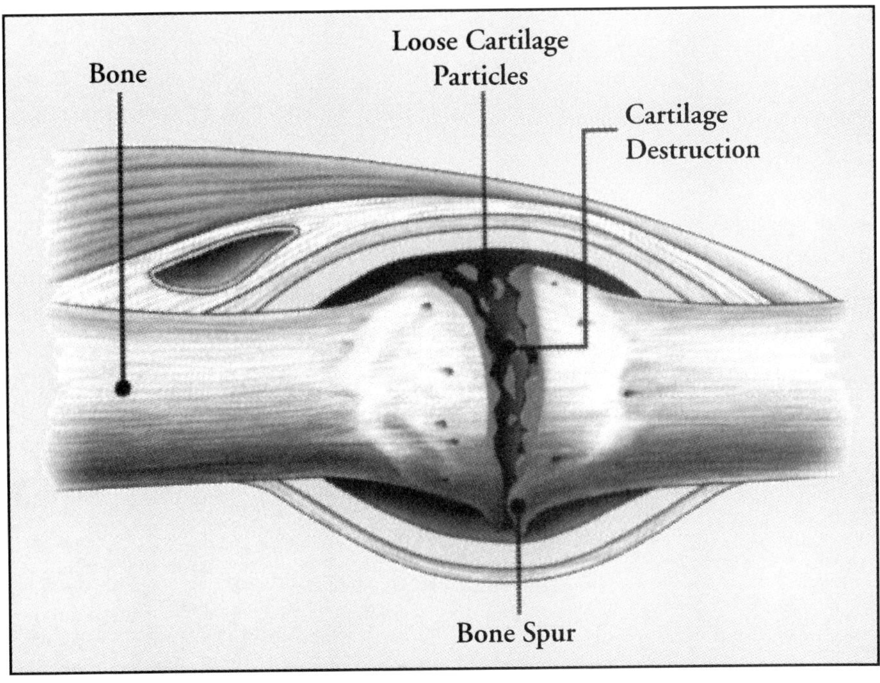

In osteoarthritis, cartilage that cushions the surface of the joint breaks down. Then the joint loses its shape and alignment, the ends of the bones thicken and form bony spurs, and bits of cartilage float in the joint space. All these changes cause pain and loss of movement.

As the damage continues, tiny pieces of cartilage and bone are shed into the synovial fluid. The synovial membrane absorbs these pieces, and becomes inflamed. This inflammation can also affect the joint capsule. In addition, ligaments may either loosen or thicken and become more rigid, which makes it hard to move the joint.[5]

Rheumatoid Arthritis

The most severe form of arthritis is rheumatoid arthritis. It is also one of the most poorly understood forms of the disease, despite extensive research.

Rheumatoid arthritis is more than just the inflammation of the joints, although that is its main symptom. The disease seems to be caused by a malfunction of the body's immune system. The immune system is supposed to help the body protect itself from disease and repair any damage. In rheumatoid arthritis, the immune system attacks healthy tissue instead, particularly the joints.

The immune system sends white blood cells, which normally seek out and destroy invading germs, into the synovial membrane. This process produces pain and swelling. In severe cases, fluid builds up in the joint, and the cells and other byproducts of the inflammation of the synovial membrane can damage the cartilage. The cartilage damage can cause the same kind of deterioration to the bone and joint capsule as osteoarthritis. Left untreated, the whole joint may break down or become deformed.[6]

Although it is mainly noticed in the joints, rheumatoid

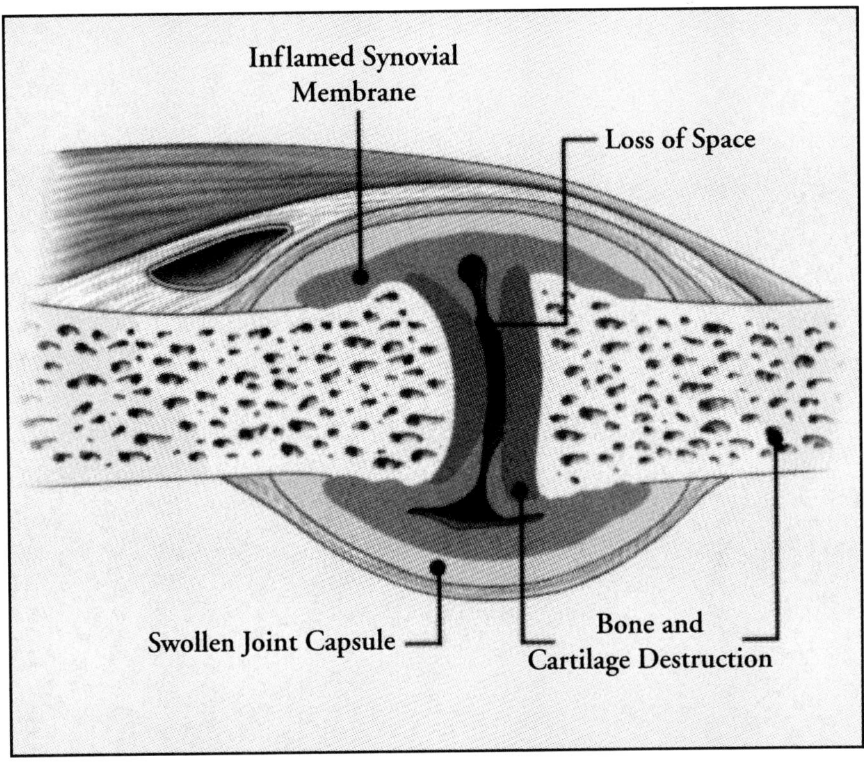

In rheumatoid arthritis, the body's own immune system attacks the joint lining, or synovial membrane. This results in the thickening of the lining. The disease can also invade and damage bone and cartilage, and the joint can lose its shape and alignment.

arthritis really attacks the entire system. Additional symptoms that are not always visible can include fatigue, low-grade fever, rashes, anemia, and dry eyes and mouth, among others. Severe cases can produce serious complications, including an inflammation of the membrane around the heart (the pericardium), scarring and thickening of lung tissue, and a buildup of fluid in the lungs.

Every patient's experience of rheumatoid arthritis is different. For some it is a mere annoyance; for others it can be crippling.

Juvenile Rheumatoid Arthritis

Juvenile rheumatoid arthritis is really a group of at least three diseases that cause inflamed joints in children under the age of sixteen. Fortunately, these diseases do not usually cause permanent joint damage or disability (although they can), and most children seem to outgrow them. Juvenile rheumatoid arthritis affects more than seventy thousand children in the United States.[7]

In addition to swollen, painful joints, symptoms of juvenile rheumatoid arthritis may include fever, anemia, and loss of appetite. In severe cases, children's growth and sexual development may be delayed.[8]

The disease can cause children to miss school and miss out on other activities with friends. It can even lead to missed career opportunities. A child with severe juvenile arthritis, for instance, is unlikely to make plans to be a forest ranger or follow some other career path that involves intense physical activity. Even playing music or creating art might seem impossible. Even if the child grows out of the disease, as many children do, it may be too late for that child to follow paths that were open to healthy children.

Most forms of juvenile rheumatoid arthritis affect more girls than boys; scientists don't know why. Although it can develop at any time, it shows up most often between the ages of one and three or in the early teenage years.[9]

Types of Juvenile Arthritis[10]

Juvenile arthritis usually follows one of three main patterns. Each behaves differently, requires a different treatment, and has a different outcome.

Systemic onset type. The initial symptoms are usually a very high fever and, often, a skin rash. Many internal organs as well as the joints may become inflamed. About 10 percent of children with arthritis have this type.

Pauciarticular onset disease. About half the children with arthritis have this type, which can strike children under age five. The condition affects fewer than five joints, but may cause eye inflammation. This disease can evolve into an adult form of arthritis in older children.

Polyarticular onset disease. This form of juvenile arthritis can begin at any age. The term is used when five or more joints (sometimes many more) are affected. Some children with this disease actually have adult-type rheumatoid arthritis that has begun much earlier than usual.

Ankylosing Spondylitis

Ankylosing spondylitis is a fairly common form of arthritis, affecting almost one in a hundred people. It is an inflammation of the joints in the spine. Unlike many forms of arthritis, it affects more men than women, usually showing up in their twenties or thirties. Although its cause is unknown, people who have a close relative with the disease are more likely to develop it themselves, which seems to indicate it might, at least partially, be inherited.[11]

The name *ankylosing spondylitis* describes what can happen in severe cases of the disease. *Ankylosing* means freezing or stiffening of a joint. *Spondylitis* is an inflammation of the joints in the spine. The disease attacks the tendons and ligaments that hold these joints together. In severe cases the tendons and ligaments can become almost as hard and calcified as bone. If that happens, the spine can become permanently locked into a stiff, unbending position. However, this happens in very few cases. Most people suffer back pain and stiffness, but are not disabled.

Gout and Pseudogout

Gout is one of the few types of arthritis for which both the cause and treatment are known.

Despite the "humors" theory of the ancient Greeks, gout is really caused by the buildup in the joint of crystals of a chemical called monosodium urate. People with gout have excessive amounts of uric acid in their blood. Uric acid is a waste product formed in the body by the breakdown of chemicals called purines. Since purines are produced naturally by the body itself and are also common in food, especially meat, uric acid is normally present in our blood to a certain degree.

Normally, our kidneys filter out excess uric acid and get rid of it in our urine. However, if the blood contains too much uric acid, crystals of the acid can settle out and be deposited inside the body. If these sharp, needle-like crystals settle in a joint, they can cause severe pain and swelling. Although doctors are not sure why, the big toe is usually affected first, followed by other joints.

Gout most often strikes men who are middle-aged or older. High blood pressure, overweight, and excessive drinking seem to contribute to its appearance. So does eating organ meats (liver, for example), which are rich in purines.[12]

Pseudogout is also caused by crystals forming in the joints. However, in pseudogout, the crystals are made of a salt called calcium pyrophosphate dihydrate (CPPD). Pseudogout is only one form of CPPD disease. CPPD disease can mimic both osteoarthritis and rheumatoid arthritis. The origin of CPPD disease is unknown.[13]

Systemic Lupus Erythematosus

Systemic lupus erythematosus, often simply called lupus, gets its name from a rash that spreads in a butterfly pattern over the bridge of the nose and cheeks of some patients, making them resemble a wolf. (*Lupus* is the Latin word for wolf.)

Like rheumatoid arthritis, lupus is a disease in which the immune system appears to attack its own body—no one knows why. It affects about one in every two thousand people. It usually strikes between the ages of twenty and forty. It is particularly common among African Americans. As well, 85 percent of its victims are women.[14]

Although lupus causes inflammation in many parts of the body, the joints almost always become inflamed, so lupus is considered a form of arthritis. However, it can also attack the skin, muscles, lymph nodes, spleen, kidneys, and other organs. In severe cases it can even be fatal.[15]

Lyme Disease and Other Infective Arthritis

Many types of arthritis are caused by infections that spread to the joints, producing inflammation. The infection can be caused by either a bacteria or a virus.

One of the most common forms of infective arthritis is Lyme disease, caused by a bacteria transmitted by a tick that feeds on deer. It was first recognized in 1975 in the town of Lyme, in southern Connecticut, where entire families were being diagnosed with a mysterious form of arthritis.[16] It took several years of research to determine that this disease was transmitted by ticks.

People infected with Lyme disease usually first suffer from fever, headache, and other flu-like symptoms. In addition, a peculiar circular rash with a bright-red border often (but not always) appears at the site of the tick bite.

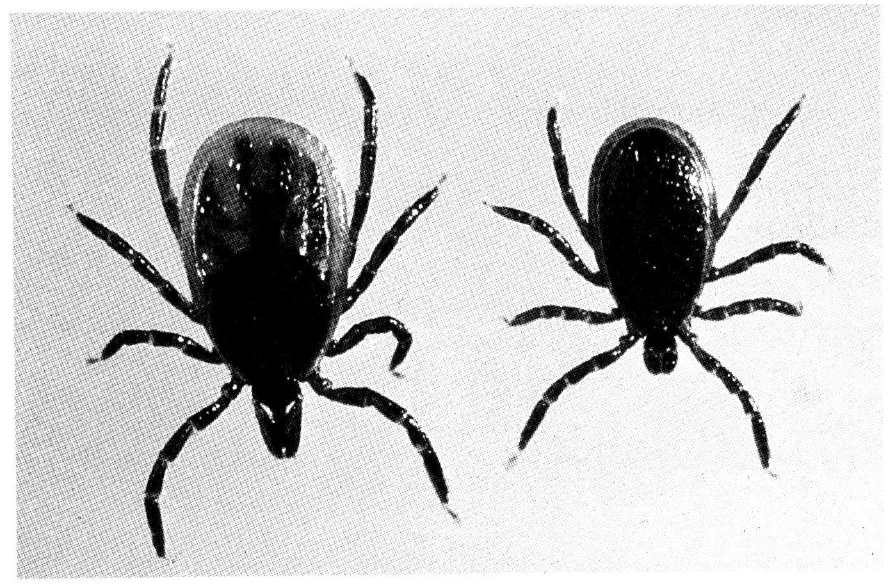

Deer ticks (*Ixodes scapularis*), enlarged here under the microscope, carry Lyme disease. It was first recognized in 1975 in Lyme, Connecticut.

The rash soon disappears, but it is followed by the second phase of the disease, which can include inflammation of the heart and nervous system, severe headache, neck pain and stiffness, meningitis, paralysis of facial muscles, and joint and muscle pains.

In the third phase of the disease, arthritis sets in, frequently affecting the knees but also involving other joints. Without treatment, this arthritis may come and go for years.

Fortunately, prompt treatment with antibiotics can stop many of the more severe symptoms of Lyme disease from developing. An even better method of prevention is to avoid getting bitten by ticks at all, by wearing long-sleeved shirts and long pants tucked into high socks when you go into a wooded area; using insect repellent that contains deet, a tick-repelling chemical; and checking carefully for ticks when you get home.

Other diseases that can produce arthritis include gonorrhea, rheumatic fever, and HIV. Other bacteria, viruses, and even fungi can cause arthritis symptoms, as well.[17]

Symptoms

In many cases, as just noted, arthritis isn't a disease at all; it's a symptom of some other disease. But whether the patient is suffering from osteoarthritis or rheumatoid arthritis, or has aching joints because of an infection or some unknown cause, the symptoms are generally the same.

Typical arthritis symptoms are swelling, redness, and warmth in a joint, restricted movement, and, of course, pain. The recommendation by the Arthritis Foundation is, "If you have pain, stiffness, or swelling in or around a joint for more than two weeks, it's time to see your doctor."[18]

Each type of arthritis has some symptoms specific to it. Rheumatoid arthritis in particular has symptoms that go beyond pain in the joints. These symptoms include mild fever; fatigue; weakness in the muscles, ligaments, tendons, and surrounding joints; and sleeplessness (as a result of pain).

The severity of symptoms varies from person to person, even among people who have the same form of arthritis.

4

Diagnosing Arthritis

Life for Doreen Belyea, age twenty-seven, looked rosy. She and her husband, Jay, had good jobs; and they had just moved into a new house in Saint John, New Brunswick, Canada, with their young family.

Then, in May 1993, the pain started. Doreen's feet would swell and cramp so badly that sometimes, if she took off her shoes, she could not put them back on again. "I went to the doctor and he told me I was wearing cheap shoes," Doreen says, but new shoes didn't help.

Soon Doreen started feeling fatigued. Then it became extremely painful to move her hip. She thought it might be a pinched nerve, but the hip kept hurting.

By September, she was in severe pain, and her hands were swelling. Finally, in November, a blood test confirmed that

Doreen had rheumatoid arthritis. "My whole life has changed," she says. "It's been devastating."[1]

As Doreen's story indicates, it is not always easy to diagnose arthritis. That is because aches and pains in joints or muscles can be caused by many different diseases, not all of which are forms of arthritis.

Diagnosing arthritis (or just about any other illness) has three main steps: providing a medical history, taking a physical examination, and having laboratory tests performed.

The Medical History

To a doctor, your medical history consists of your own description of your current symptoms and how they came about, plus a complete review of any other medical problems you have now or have had in the past, in addition to such basic information as your age, gender, activities, etc. The more the doctor knows about you, the better he or she can determine what is wrong with you and how that condition will affect your everyday life.

People who are suffering from arthritis most commonly complain of joint pain or stiffness (although they may also suffer from symptoms such as fatigue, fever, headache, and weight loss), so much of the medical history the doctor gathers will focus on the joints.

Typical questions the doctor might ask include which joints hurt, when and how the pain started, how it spread from joint to joint (if it has), what makes the pain begin, what makes it feel better, what time of the day it is at its worst, whether any joints lock or give way, and if the patient is stiff in the morning.

Once those questions are answered, the doctor has a better idea of what kind of arthritis the patient might have. Then he or she can move on to more specific questions designed to try to pin down the exact type of arthritis. For example, if the doctor suspects lupus, he or she might ask about skin rashes or chest pains; if the doctor suspects ankylosing spondylitis, he or she might ask about back pains or eye problems.

Once the patient's medical history is established, the doctor can move on to a physical examination.

The Physical Examination

The physical examination actually begins the moment the doctor sees the patient. "I like to watch the way a patient gets out of a chair and walks toward my examining room," says David S. Pisetsky, chief of rheumatology at the Durham, North Carolina, Veterans Administration Hospital. "Does he appear comfortable in a sitting position or when rising? Does he limp? When he gestures or moves, does he look as if he is in pain? By watching these actions, I can learn a great deal about the nature of his joint pain."[2]

As part of the physical examination, the doctor checks blood pressure, pulse rate, heart, and lungs before concentrating on the joints. The doctor looks to see how many joints are involved, if the same joints on both sides of the body are affected, which joints are involved (large, small, or both), and whether the spine is also affected.

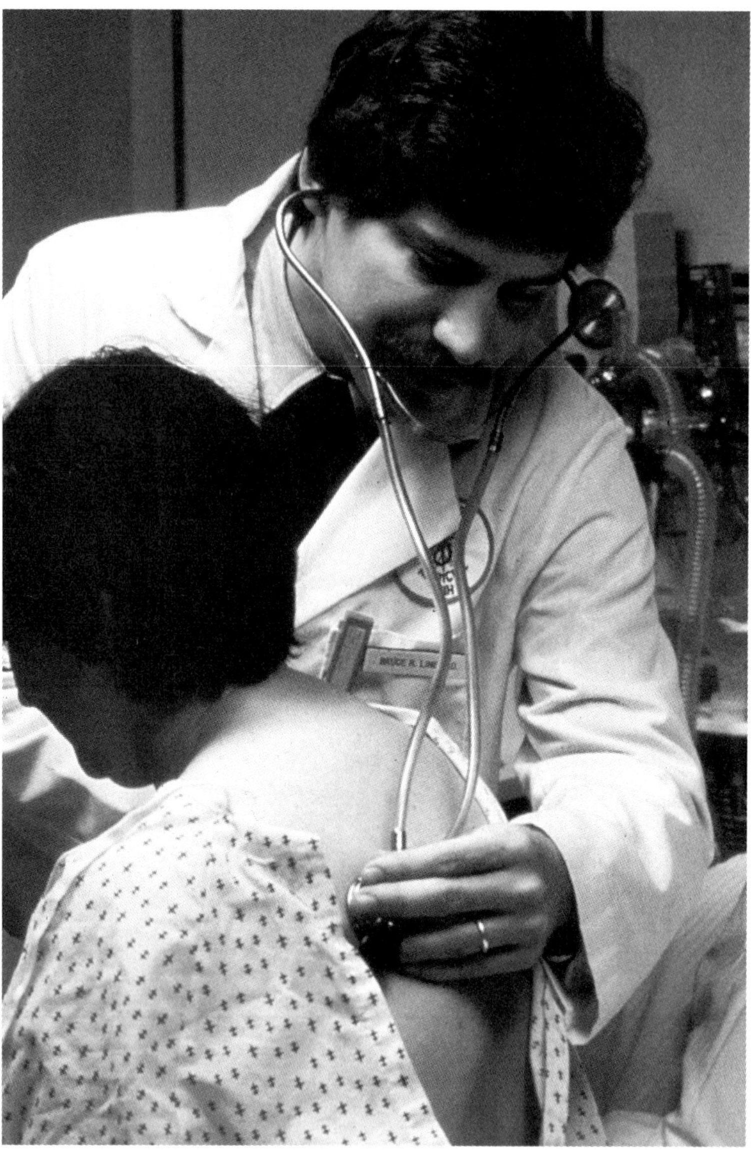

A doctor examines a patient to determine whether she has arthritis, and if so, what type. Along with examining the patient's joints, the doctor will check the patient's blood pressure, pulse rate, and other vital signs.

The doctor tries to determine how much movement of the joints has been limited and also looks for any deformities. At the same time, he or she looks for other physical signs, such as the type of rashes that lupus can cause or the painless lumps that sometimes appear under the skin in patients with rheumatoid arthritis.

With the physical examination completed, the doctor is in a position to order laboratory tests.

Laboratory Tests for Arthritis

By the time the doctor has finished taking a medical history and performing a physical examination, he or she probably has a pretty good idea of what type of arthritis a patient may have. Laboratory tests can back up the doctor's opinion and point the way to the best treatment.

Blood tests. The most common type of laboratory test is a blood test. That's because blood is the easiest and safest tissue in the body to sample, and contains traces of material from every other part of the body.

The most basic blood test is called a complete blood count, or CBC. Blood consists of red blood cells, white blood cells, and platelets, all suspended in a colorless fluid called plasma. The number of red and white cells and platelets can be quickly counted by a machine. If joints are inflamed, the red blood cell count may be low (anemia is the official name of this condition), and the white blood cell and platelet count may be high.[3]

Another test for inflammation is called the erythrocyte sedimentation rate, or "sed rate," for short. Whenever blood is left standing in a test tube, the red blood cells in it gradually settle to the bottom of the tube. The distance the red blood cells fall in one hour is the sed rate. In blood from someone who is healthy, the rate is about twenty millimeters per hour; in blood from someone who is suffering from an inflammation, the rate can be more than five times faster.[4]

Meanwhile, the plasma can also be analyzed to see what it contains. These analytic tests are called "chemistries." For example, the amount of uric acid in the plasma can be measured. The majority of gout patients have high levels of this acid in their blood.[5]

Another substance doctors look for in the blood is called the "rheumatoid factor." When bacteria, viruses, and other invaders enter the body, the body's immune system creates substances called antibodies to fight these outside organisms. Each antibody is designed specifically to combat a particular type of invader. In diseases such as lupus, however, the immune system forms antibodies to attack the body itself. Rheumatoid factor is one of these self-attacking types of antibodies. It is found in about 80 percent of people who are suffering from rheumatoid arthritis.[6]

Similarly, patients with lupus have antibodies to DNA, the substance contained in all cells that serves as a blueprint for the next generation of cells. Very few people without lupus have this antibody, so this is a particularly useful blood test for diagnosing that disease.[7]

There are many other blood tests that can be performed, but these are some of the most common.

Other Tests. There are several other standard types of laboratory tests that the doctor may order. One is a urine test, in which a sample of the patient's urine is examined to see what it contains. Lupus and some other rheumatic diseases may cause kidney damage. This can result in the presence of red blood cells, protein, or other substances that are not normally found in the urine.[8]

Sometimes the doctor may carry out a joint fluid test. In this test, a needle is inserted into a joint and some of the synovial fluid is removed. This procedure sounds painful, but it is generally no more so than drawing blood. Examining the fluid may show what is causing the problem, or at least what is not causing the problem. If the synovial fluid is clear and contains few white blood cells, the joint is not considered inflamed, and the only type of arthritis it might be considered to display is osteoarthritis. If the fluid is cloudy and contains a lot of white blood cells, the joint is definitely inflamed. If it contains crystals, the patient is suffering from gout, and if bacteria are present, the joint is considered infected.[9]

Another basic laboratory test is an X ray, which lets the doctor see exactly what is happening inside the joint. X rays are particularly useful in helping the doctor tell the difference between osteoarthritis and rheumatoid arthritis.

In osteoarthritis, the space between the bones in a joint is narrower than it should be and uneven. The bones may also thicken and develop spurs, or osteocytes. In rheumatoid arthritis, however, the joint space narrows evenly, tissue swells, and bones around the joint become less dense.[10]

By combining the results of all of these lab tests with the doctor's own observations and the patient's medical history, the doctor will usually feel confident in diagnosing what type of arthritis the patient has.

Then, of course, it is time to sit down and talk about types of treatment.

5

Treatment of Arthritis

After he spent one summer working for a building contractor, Jim, a twenty-year-old college student, began to notice a nagging pain and stiffness in his lower back. It was most severe in the morning, but got better as the day went along.

Jim was sure he had hurt himself at work, but he couldn't figure out how. He tried using a heating pad on his sore back, but that didn't help. He went to a chiropractor, but that did not help, either. A local doctor gave him drugs to relax his muscles. These helped to ease the pain, but they did not make the pain go away.

Jim began to worry that the pain would interfere with his upcoming studies and sports, so he went to see an orthopedic surgeon. X rays showed changes in the joints in his lower spine, so he was sent on to a rheumatology clinic, where he was diagnosed with ankylosing spondylitis.

The rheumatologist prescribed a drug designed to reduce inflammation and started Jim on a program of physical therapy. He also told Jim to take it easy until his back felt better.

When school started, Jim was able to carry out all his regular activities, including sports. The rule, the doctor said, was to live normally as long as he felt OK—but the doctor couldn't promise that he would always feel OK.

Jim's story is typical. For most forms of arthritis, there is no cure. Instead, the goal is to manage the symptoms so that the patient can continue to live a near-normal life.

Jim's treatment was typical, too. The basic elements of all arthritis treatments are rest, exercise, and drugs. For some forms of arthritis, surgery can also help.

It might sound contradictory that doctors tell patients to both rest and exercise. However, as in Jim's case, the goal is to rest and relax when the pain is bad, then exercise when the pain is less acute.

Rest

Pain is the body's way of telling us that something is wrong—that we've injured ourselves or are about to, for instance, or that we have picked up an infection. In arthritis, pain is primarily the result of inflammation and damage to the affected joints. Pain can also result from muscle tension. By protecting sore joints, arthritis patients may overexert muscles they don't normally use.[1]

Goals of Treatment[2]

For most forms of arthritis, there is no cure. Instead, treatment has these more modest, but still important, goals:

- Relieve pain
- Reduce inflammation
- Slow down or stop damage to the joints
- Improve a person's sense of well-being and ability to function

Many forms of arthritis flare up, or become more acute, from time to time. During these "flares," rest is particularly important. For example, patients with rheumatoid arthritis find that there are times when their joints are warmer, more swollen, and more painful than other times. When that happens, a period of rest helps settle the disease and reduce the inflammation. Rheumatoid arthritis and lupus patients often find they fatigue easily, too; resting regularly allows them to conserve energy.

Exercise

However, even when patients are resting, it's important that they also exercise. Doing nothing weakens muscles and allows the joints to stiffen, making it harder, not easier, to get around. Exercise keeps joints mobile. It also improves one's overall level of fitness, reduces stress, and promotes healthy sleep patterns—which, in turn, reduce fatigue.

Range-of-motion exercises to build flexibility are particularly important, even when the arthritis has flared up (although painful joints should be moved gently). Range-of-motion exercises aim to gently move each joint as far as possible in all directions. Done daily, these exercises help keep joints fully mobile and prevent stiffness and deformities.

Strengthening and endurance exercises are also recommended, but not during flares. Maintaining muscle strength is important because strong muscles help support and protect

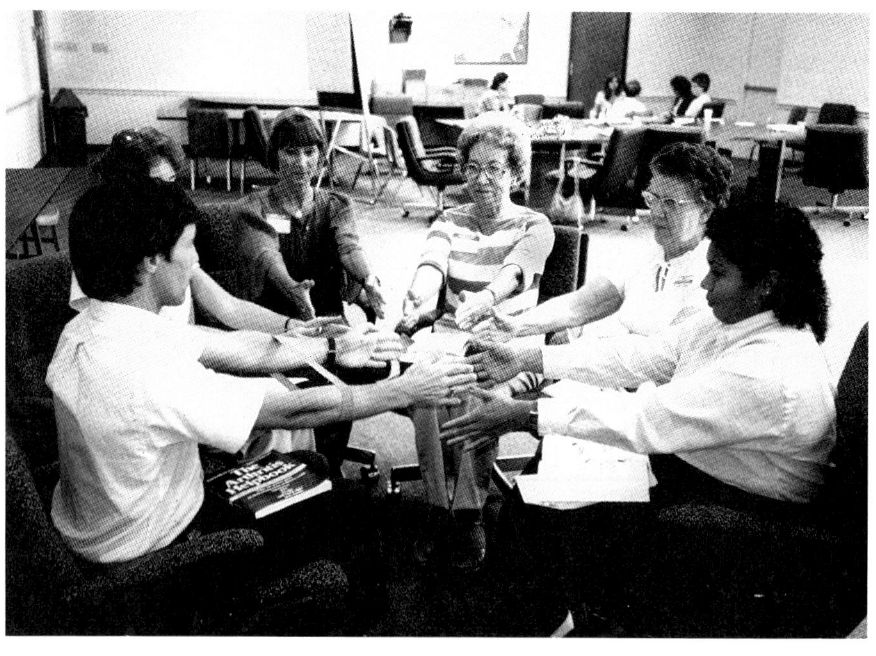

Range-of-motion exercises specially designed for arthritis sufferers can help them maintain full use of their joints.

joints. Several studies have also shown that improving muscle strength decreases pain.[3] Endurance exercises, which raise the heart rate for an extended period of time, are important for overall fitness.

All exercises have to be carefully tailored to the individual patient to insure that they work the right muscles but don't overstress arthritic joints.

Medications

Many different types of medications are prescribed for arthritis, but they generally fall into one of two categories:

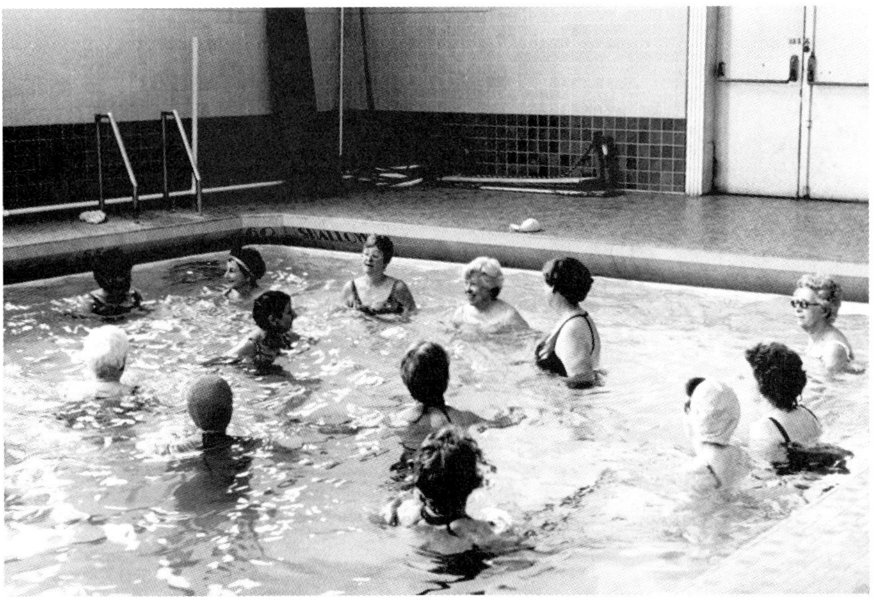

Water aerobics and other water exercises typically put less stress on the joints than other types of exercises. Because water supports some of the body's weight and provides resistance to movement, exercising in water is good therapy for people with arthritis.

anti-inflammatory drugs and disease-modifying drugs. Some patients take both.

Anti-inflammatory drugs reduce inflammation in the joints. Most of them work by slowing the body's production of an enzyme called cyclooxygenase. Reducing cyclooxygenase in the body also reduces the body's production of other substances called prostaglandins, which play a key role in inflammation. Prostaglandins work by dilating, or opening up, blood vessels, allowing an increased blood flow to the inflamed area (which creates redness and swelling). In addition, prostaglandins interact with other substances released during inflammation to cause pain and fever. They also appear indirectly to promote the weakening of the bone and cartilage.[4] Therefore, by reducing the body's production of prostaglandins, anti-inflammatory drugs are able to reduce the effects of inflammation.

The most basic and common anti-inflammatory drug is acetylsalicylic acid, or aspirin, which has been in use for more than a hundred years. In addition to reducing inflammation, it also helps relieve pain.

Many other nonsteroidal anti-inflammatory drugs, or NSAIDs, work in much the same way as aspirin. Many NSAIDs, like aspirin, can be bought without a prescription. They include ibuprofen, naproxen sodium, and ketoprofen.[5] Others can be obtained only with a prescription.

NSAIDs can cause unpleasant side effects. That's because prostaglandins, which are diminished by taking NSAIDs, don't just contribute to inflammation; they also protect the

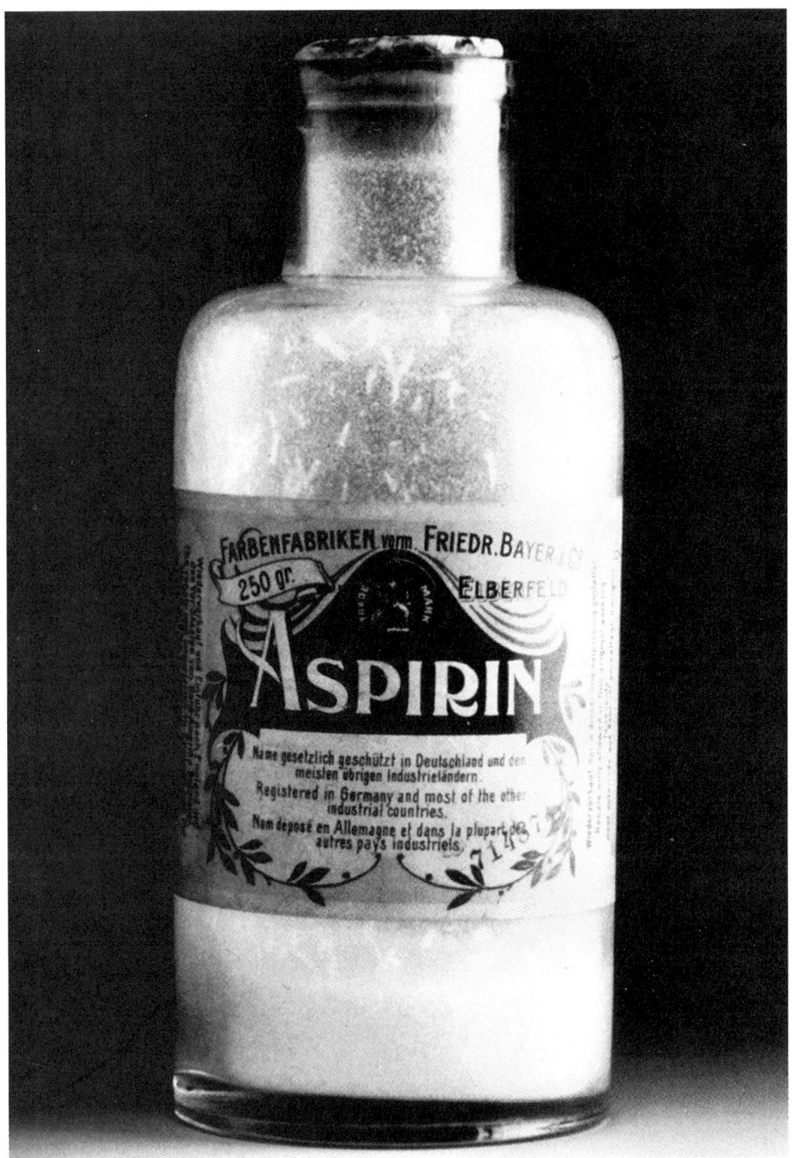

This is the first bottle of aspirin. The drug was manufactured and distributed in powder form by the Bayer Company in Germany beginning in 1899.

stomach lining, promote blood clotting, and regulate salt and fluid balance. As a result, stomach irritation, bleeding, fluid retention, and decreased kidney function sometimes result from taking NSAIDs.[6]

Recently, some new types of NSAIDs have become available. Collectively called Cox-2 inhibitors, these drugs work as well as the older NSAIDs, but don't have the same gastrointestinal side effects. That's because the body produces two different types of cyclooxygenase, Cox-1 and Cox-2. The older NSAIDs block Cox-1, which is also responsible for protecting our gastrointestinal tract.[7] The new drugs block Cox-2 instead, avoiding the problems caused by blocking Cox-1.

One of the first Cox-2 inhibitors on the market is called Celebrex™; others are currently being tested.[8]

When more powerful anti-inflammatory drugs are required, doctors turn to corticosteroids, synthetic versions of the hormone cortisol. Cortisol is normally produced by the outer layer of the adrenal glands. (Remember, NSAIDs are *nonsteroidal* anti-inflammatory drugs. That is to distinguish them from the cortico*steroids*.) Corticosteroids were developed in 1948 and seemed, at the time, the next best thing to a cure for arthritis. However, as time went by, serious side effects were noted, such as weight gain, high blood pressure, osteoporosis (a weakening of the bones), cataracts, and ulcers. Today corticosteroids are administered much more cautiously, but they can still be of great benefit.

Cortisol, the hormone corticosteroids are based on, helps control the salt and water balance in the body and the use of

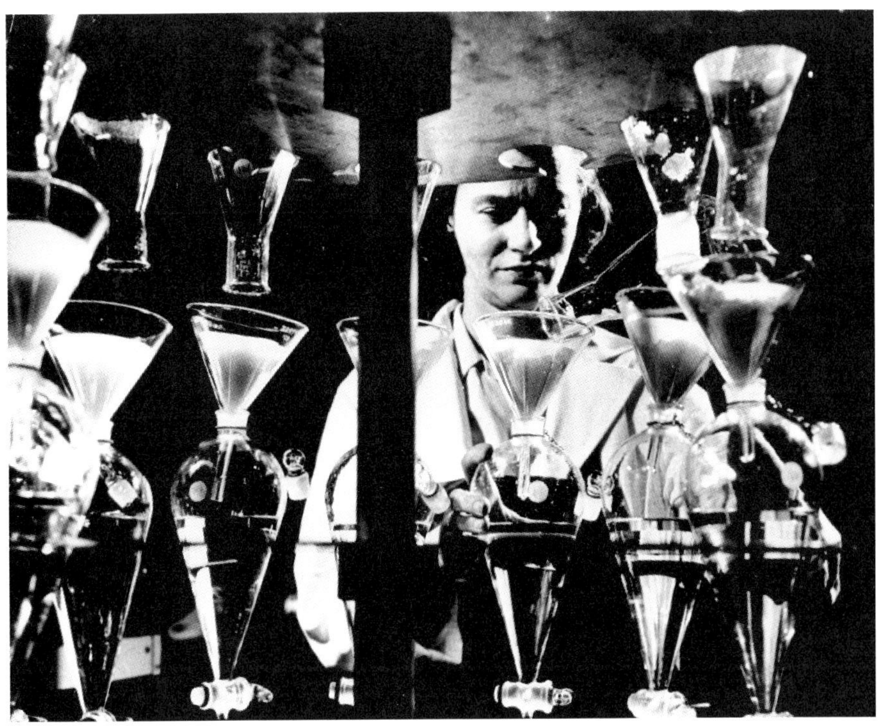

A researcher attempts to isolate cortisol and related hormones during the 1950s. Today many synthesized corticosteroids have been proven to have serious side effects.

the carbohydrates, fat, and protein in our food. When we're under stress or are hurt, more cortisol is naturally released. Anyone who has played a contact sport has experienced the effects of extra cortisol. While you're playing, you don't feel any pain, even after crashing into other players. Afterward, however, you may feel stiff and sore, as the stress and excitement go away.

Corticosteroids, like NSAIDs, block the productio substances like prostaglandins that trigger inflamma

However, they can make white blood cells work less efficiently, which makes the body more susceptible to infection.[9]

The most commonly prescribed corticosteroid for arthritis is prednisone, which is four to five times as strong as cortisone. It comes in tablet form.[10]

Disease-modifying drugs slow the disease process in the forms of arthritis caused by the immune system attacking the body, such as rheumatoid arthritis and lupus. Not all drugs work with all patients, so their use has to be closely monitored. It sometimes takes weeks or months to find out if a particular drug is doing any good. Because they are very strong and may have unpleasant side effects, they are usually tried only after NSAIDs have failed to control the arthritis.

One interesting disease-modifying drug is gold salts, which have been used for sixty years. Nobody knows why they work. Like many medical breakthroughs, they were discovered by accident. A French physician named Jacques Forrestier was researching a theory that metals could treat infections. When he injected gold salts into some tuberculosis patients who also had arthritis, their arthritis began to improve, although, unfortunately, their tuberculosis did not.[11]

Another disease-modifying drug is penicillamine. Although it is related to penicillin, it has different effects. Again, nobody is sure why it works, but it may stop certain types of white blood cells from causing joint damage.[12]

Another drug sometimes used to treat rheumatoid arthritis is hydroxychloroquine. This drug was originally developed to treat malaria. It is useful in some cases of lupus as well as rheumatoid arthritis. Again, no one is entirely sure why or how it works.[13]

None of these drugs, nor any of the many others that are sometimes used to treat arthritis, is effective in all patients. Penicillamine and hydroxychloroquine work in about 30 percent of cases, while gold salts seem to work well in about 10 percent of cases and provide some benefit in 40 to 50 percent.[14]

Drug therapy often has to be readjusted as the disease progresses. Often, patients find that the first time they're given a new drug, it helps them a lot. As time goes on, however, it helps them less and less. As a result, the doctor may prescribe a series of different drugs.

No one is certain why arthritis drugs often lose their effectiveness over time. One possibility is that some drugs stimulate the liver to produce more of the enzymes it uses routinely to try to render toxins harmless. These enzymes can also neutralize the effectiveness of the drugs being taken.[15]

Surgery

Surgery is usually a last resort in treating arthritis, and is only used for patients with severe joint damage. There are several different types of surgery that can be beneficial.

Arthroscopy is the viewing of the inside of a joint. To do so, doctors use a fine tube with a tiny lens attached to it. The tube is inserted into the joint through a small incision. While the tube is in the joint, the surgeon can use fine tools on the tube's end to remove material or fluid for further examination, carry out repairs on torn cartilage or ligaments, or even shave the kneecap smooth. Arthroscopy is often performed on people suffering from osteoarthritis, to see the exact condition of the affected joint.[16]

Arthrodesis is another type of operation sometimes performed. This procedure fuses the bones in a joint together. Afterward, the joint can't bend anymore, but the procedure can correct deformity and make unstable joints more stable. In general, during this operation the cartilage from the ends of the bones is removed, and the surface layer of the bones is shaved away; then the bones are drawn together and held in place by screws, plates, or rods. Eventually new bone grows and fuses the two pieces of bone together. This procedure is commonly performed on joints of the hands, feet, ankles, hips, and spine, among others.

Joint replacement surgery is performed to relieve pain and improve joint function and appearance. In joint replacement surgery, the diseased joint is removed and replaced with an artificial one made of polyethylene (a very tough plastic) and metal alloy. Knees and hips are the most commonly replaced joints. Replacement joints are themselves not permanent, and after about ten years sometimes have to be replaced.[17]

Tendon reconstruction surgery rebuilds a damaged tendon by attaching an intact one to it. (Rheumatoid arthritis can damage tendons, which attach muscle to bone, especially in the hands.) This procedure can restore or preserve some hand function, particularly if it is done before a tendon breaks completely.[18] In a slightly different operation, a tendon that has

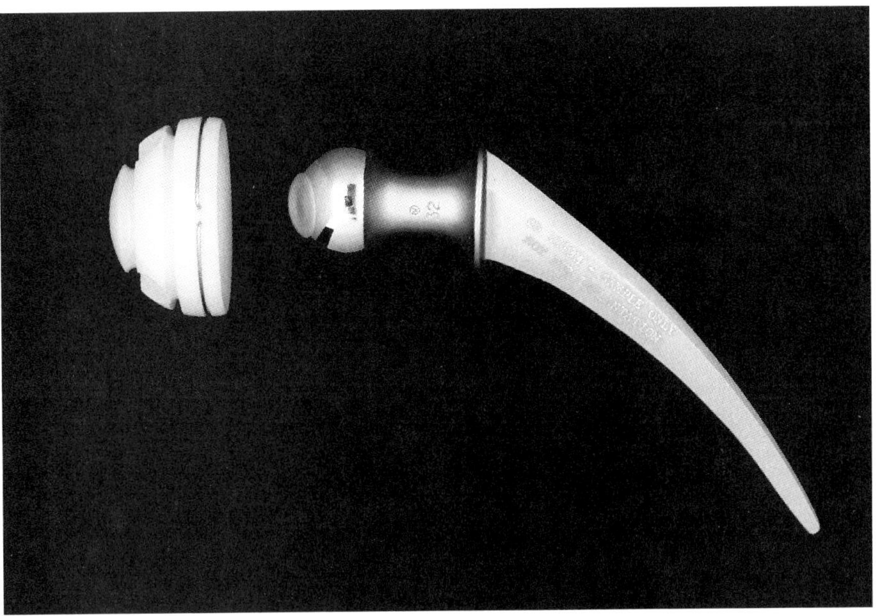

Hip joints are commonly replaced by artificial joints made of tough plastic and metal alloy. The right-hand part of this synthetic joint is the ball, which swivels inside the socket on the left.

contracted, restricting movement and sometimes causing pain, may be released.

Synovectomy is most commonly performed on a knee. The doctor removes the inflamed synovial membrane. Today this procedure is usually only done as part of tendon reconstruction, because the synovial membrane can't be completely removed and thus tends to grow back.[19]

Osteotomy is an operation, usually performed on the knee, in which a bone is cut. This could be to make the bone longer or shorter, or to change its alignment. Realigning bones with an osteotomy can sometimes reduce wear and tear on a joint.

An osteotomy not only relieves pain, it can sometimes stop or reverse the damage caused by osteoarthritis.[20]

Alternative Medicine

Over the years, many other alternative approaches for treating arthritis have been tried. These range from following special diets and taking vitamin supplements and various herbal remedies to remedies as bizarre as burial in horse manure, smearing brake fluid on the skin, and eating raisins previously soaked in gin.

One popular remedy is the wearing of a copper bracelet, a treatment that dates back thousands of years. Many arthritis sufferers swear copper bracelets—as well as other alternative treatments—reduce their pain. Although there is some scientific evidence to prove that copper-related substances may reduce inflammation when taken internally, there are no scientific reasons to support the belief that wearing a copper bracelet can affect the symptoms of arthritis.[21]

Some people swear that wearing magnets helps control their arthritis. The belief that magnets have healing properties dates back to the nineteenth century. Today, orthopedic surgeons use pulsed electromagnets to help speed healing in broken bones, and a great deal of research is being done into other uses for powerful magnetic fields. However, the small magnets usually worn by arthritis sufferers are many times weaker than the electromagnets researchers are studying. Most doctors believe that they simply aren't powerful enough to have any effect at all; nevertheless, a few very small-scale research projects have indicated that the magnets might have some effect on pain.[22] More research still needs to be done.

Another common alternative therapy is chiropractic treatment. Chiropractors treat disease by manipulating, or moving, the spine and other body structures. These manipulations are based on the belief that diseases are caused by pressure, especially of the vertebrae, on nerves. While chiropractors do seem to provide pain relief for some people, they cannot cure arthritis any more than regular doctors can.

Another pain-relieving alternative therapy is acupuncture. Practiced by the Chinese for more than twenty-five hundred years, acupuncture involves inserting thin needles into very specific points on the body. While the procedure does seem to relieve pain in some people, it, too, cannot offer a genuine cure for arthritis or other serious illnesses.

Acupuncture isn't the only popular alternative treatment in use for centuries. For example, creams made from a variety of herbs have been applied to the skin for thousands of years, since the time of the Babylonians, but recent studies show no real scientific benefit from such treatments.[23]

Whereas many alternative therapies, whether they work or not, are at least harmless, some herbal remedies can be dangerous. After all, many of our most powerful drugs were first identified in and synthesized from herbs. A few years ago some people claimed a Chinese herbal remedy known as *chuifong toukuwan* could relieve arthritis. Laboratory analysis of the substance found that it contained several highly dangerous

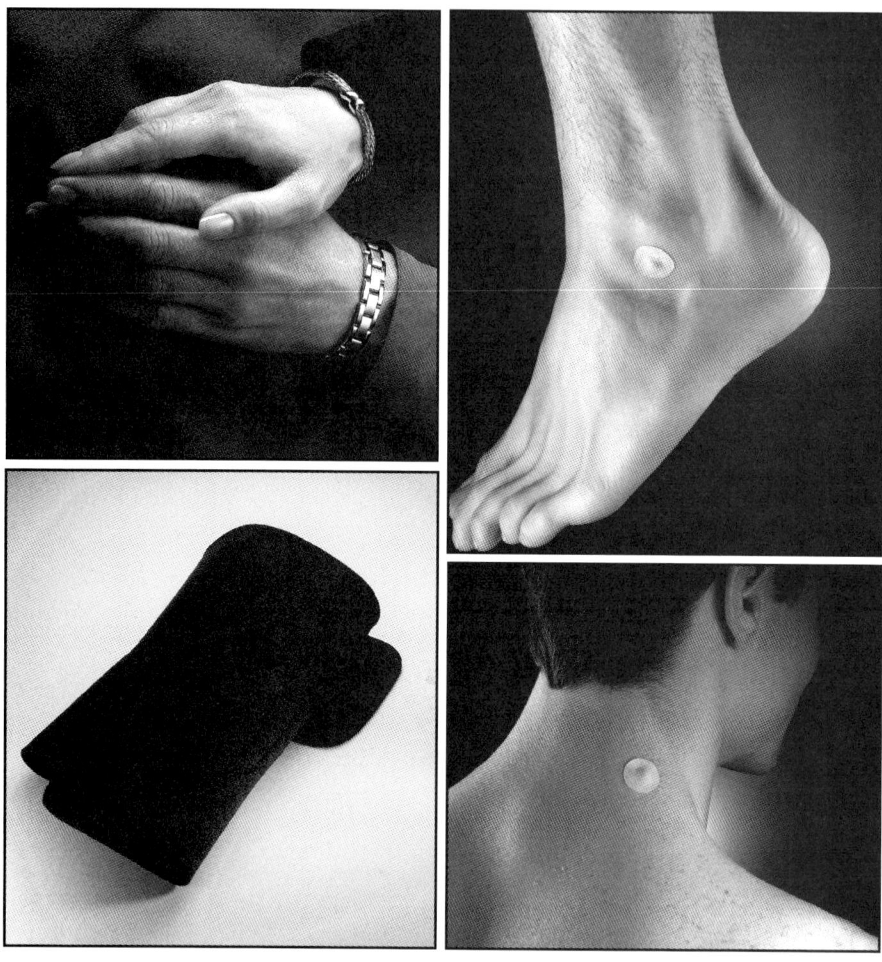

New devices using magnets are selling widely. Although the benefits of magnets have not been scientifically proven, they promise relief from arthritis pain in the joints of the back, shoulders, neck, hips, wrists, hands, elbows, ankles, and knees.

drugs, including cortisone, which doctors have learned to use with utmost caution.[24]

Another example of a potentially dangerous herbal treatment is alfalfa. Promoted in the early 1980s as a miracle "all natural" cure, alfalfa, taken in pill form or eaten naturally as sprouts, actually contains a toxin that can produce symptoms in humans similar to lupus. In other words, eating excessive amounts of alfalfa to try to improve one form of arthritis can actually cause some people to develop another.[25]

Special diets and foods thought to help arthritis sufferers have been touted for years: Honey and vinegar, pokeberries,

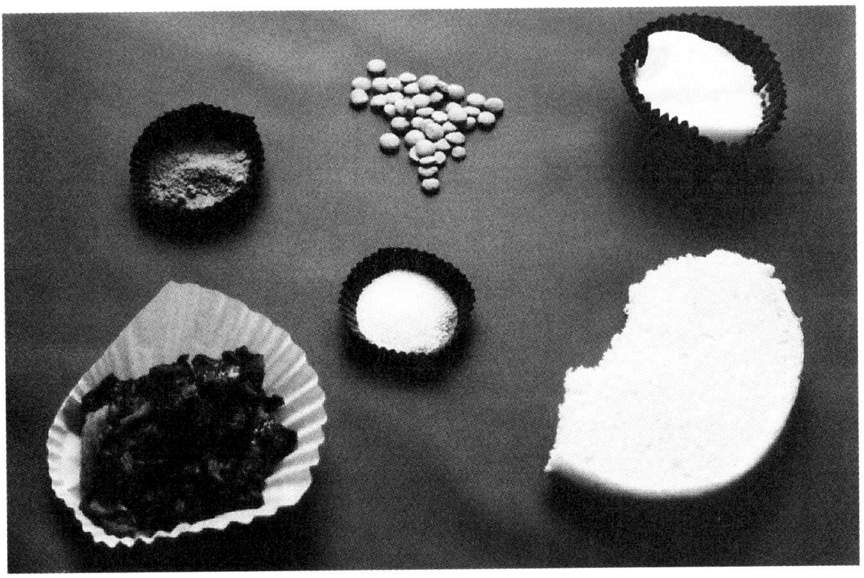

East Indian practitioners of Ayurvedic medicine use food from six basic taste groups to correct perceived imbalances in the body. Examples of the groups are (clockwise from lower left): bitter—green leafy vegetables like spinach; pungent—cumin and other spices; astringent or dry—lentils; sour—yogurt; sweet—breads; salty—salt and salty foods.

blackstrap molasses, cranberry juice, and fish oils have all been promoted as remedies. While there is some evidence that diet can influence many forms of arthritis, most of the diets promoted in the media as helpful for arthritics have not been scientifically tested.

Some people claim that eating certain foods can cause their arthritis to flare up. Although there is a proven link between diet and gout, scientific evidence of a link between specific foods and flare-ups of other types of arthritis is lacking. However, it is certainly possible that particular individuals may experience a sensitivity to certain foods that influences the course of their disease.

It is estimated that for every dollar spent on scientific research into arthritis each year, North Americans spend twenty-five dollars on unproven and dubious remedies.[26] Why are so many people willing to try them?

"Frustration. Desperation," says Dr. Richard S. Panush, an immunologist at Saint Barnabus Medical Center in Livingston, New Jersey. "Many rheumatologic diseases are chronic [incurable], and in many instances, we can't provide patients with the kind of symptomatic relief they'd like to achieve. I think in many instances, out of frustration and, in a sense, desperation, they'll look elsewhere, outside conventional medicine, for relief."

Many doctors are concerned that even if an unconventional treatment is harmless, pursuing it may lead a patient to neglect conventional treatment. That would be a shame, Panush says. "There are enormous things we can do for patients. The concern is, in a patient trying Dr. X's Magic Cure, we lose the chance to do those things we can do. . . ."[27]

Although there is still no cure for most forms of arthritis, there are many more treatments available than there have ever been before. In fact, today 90 percent of those diagnosed with arthritis can expect to "go to work, get a full night's sleep, exercise, and even participate in sports," says Lynn Gerber, chief of rehabilitation medicine at the National Institutes of Health.[28]

There are hopes for even better treatments in the near future.

6

Arthritis and Society

Arthritis has been disabling people for a very long time, and every time it strikes another individual, it also has an impact on society. That impact is felt both on a small, immediate scale and on a large, societal one.

On the small scale, there is a direct impact on the family of the patient. Nina, a woman now in her early seventies, developed rheumatoid arthritis when she was in her thirties. At various times over the years, she ended up in the hospital, for everything from nosebleeds that wouldn't stop, caused by taking large doses of aspirin, to two complete knee replacements. Although she has managed her disease well, arthritis has still taken its toll, causing her to lose days at work and putting additional stress on her family.

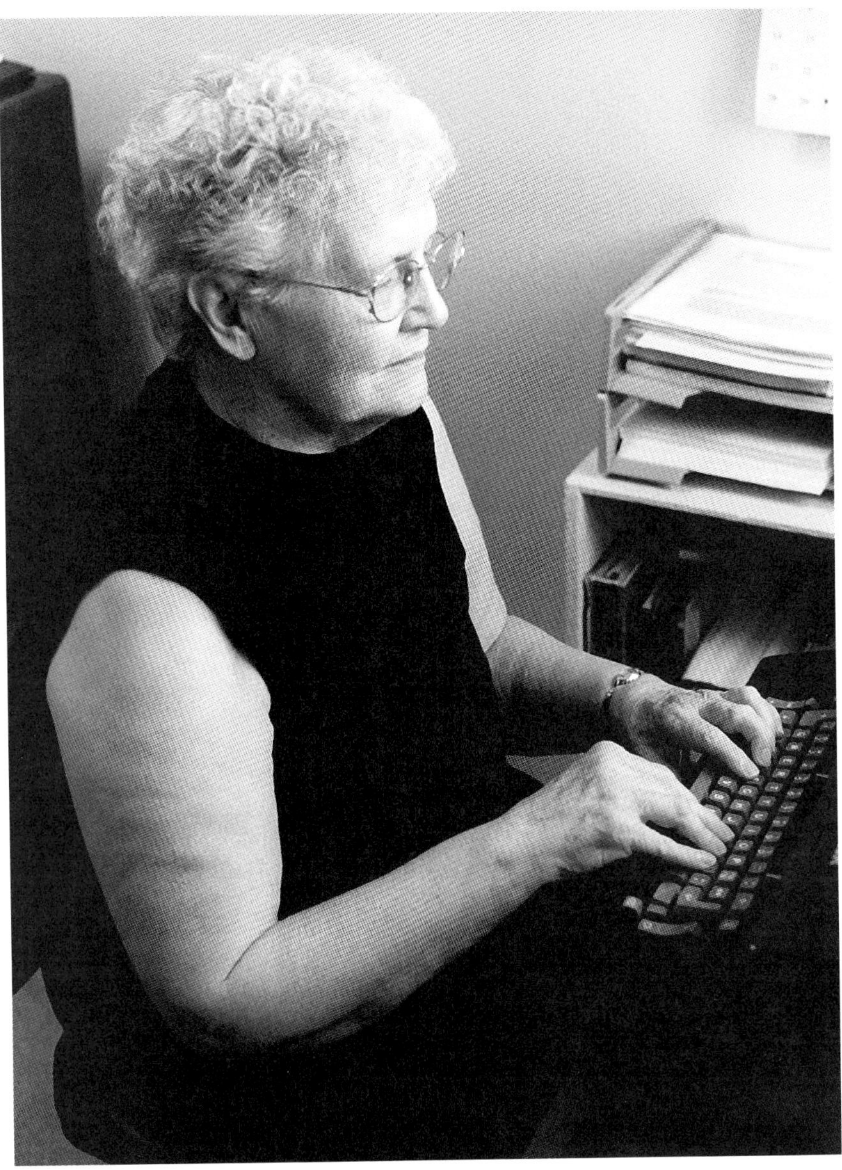

The author's mother is pictured here on a better day at her typewriter. Years ago, she was a secretary and missed many days of work due to inflammation of her fingers.

Stories like this one are repeated in family after family. "Chronic illness impacts a person's entire lifestyle—work, family and recreation," says Gail Wright, a rehabilitation psychologist at the University of Missouri, Columbia.[1] In fact, after pain, emotional problems such as anger and depression are among the most common symptoms of arthritis.[2]

One in Six

According to the Arthritis Foundation, 43 million Americans have one of the approximately one hundred different types of arthritis. That is roughly one out of every six Americans.[3] This statistic could also be interpreted to mean that one in every three families includes someone, old or young, afflicted with some form of arthritis.[4]

Another way to calculate the prevalence of arthritis is to see it in terms of odds: that is, how likely is a particular person to get arthritis? Figured that way, the risk of a child under the age of fifteen developing juvenile arthritis is about one in a thousand. For adults between the ages of thirty and fifty, the odds of developing rheumatoid arthritis are about one in one hundred. For adults over fifty, the risk of developing osteoarthritis rises to one in ten; by age sixty-five, the odds are one in four. Over age seventy-five, the odds rise to one in two.

What this statistic means is that if arthritis hasn't already affected you, it's very likely that it will. Even if you don't develop arthritis yourself, someone you know—a parent, an aunt, a brother—probably will.

The overall percentage of people suffering from arthritis will probably go up in the next few years, too. That's because the baby boomers—the enormous number of children born after World War II—are entering their fifties, the age when the risk of osteoarthritis starts to rise. As the percentage of older people in the overall population increases, so will the percentage of people with arthritis. It is estimated that the number of people suffering some form of disability resulting from osteoarthritis will be twice as high in the year 2021 as it was in 1986, and the total number of people suffering from some form of arthritis will rise to 59 million.[5]

That increase is going to mean a huge demand for the services of doctors—both family doctors and specialists—as well as those of nurses, social workers, physical therapists, and others, including the caretaking children and grandchildren of the sufferers. Because the general adult population won't be growing as fast as the elderly population, there could be a shortage of these caregivers.

Huge Financial Impact

Osteoarthritis is the leading cause of disability in the United States. Almost everyone over the age of seventy-five is affected in at least one joint.[6] The prevalence of arthritis puts a huge strain on the nation's health system.

Beyond the personal impact, arthritis has a severe financial impact on society. Back in 1923, the first survey to measure the social and economic impact of rheumatoid arthritis was conducted in Sweden. The following year another study was conducted in England. The English study revealed that a sixth of lost work time in industry was due to "rheumatism and arthritis."[7] Current American statistics indicate that osteoarthritis alone accounts for more than seven million visits to doctors per year and 36 billion work days lost.[8]

In financial terms, the direct and indirect costs of rheumatoid arthritis alone are estimated to have reached $65 billion in 1992.[9] Figure in all the other types of arthritis, and the cost is much higher.

Direct costs include hospitalization, surgery, various therapies, chronic care, home care, medical consultations, drugs, braces, aids for mobility (canes, walkers, wheelchairs, etc.), aids for daily living, and changes to homes and vehicles.

Indirect costs include days lost from work, lower productivity at work, complications from the disease, complications from treatments for arthritis (drug side effects, for instance), and the impact on the productivity of other members of the sufferer's family.[10]

Disability in all its forms has had a major impact on society. Throughout the twentieth century, there has been an ongoing battle to ensure that disabled people are able to enjoy the same access to buildings and public services as those who are not disabled. As a result, it is very rare today to see a building without a wheelchair ramp, an elevator, and several parking spaces set aside for disabled, or handicapped, people. A milestone of the fight for equal rights for disabled people was the passage of the Americans with Disabilities Act in 1990, which made many of these changes mandatory.

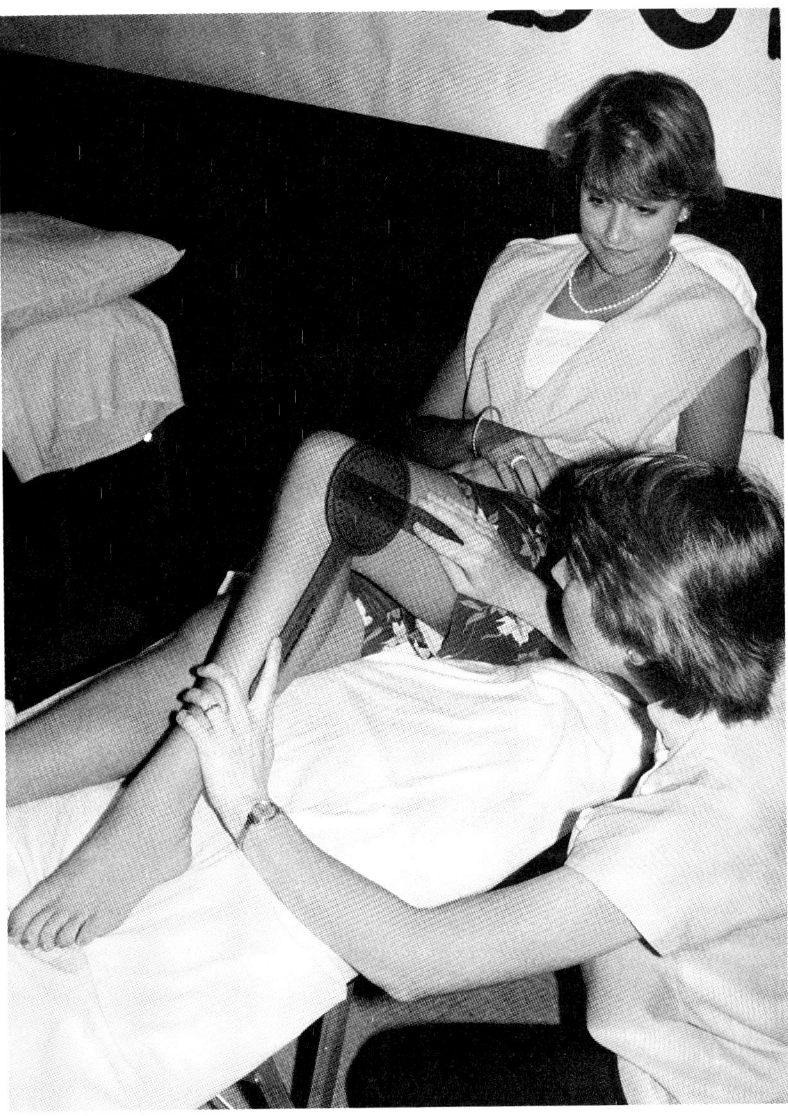

A therapist measures the range of motion in the patient's knee to see how well her therapy is helping. Therapies to help achieve greater mobility in the joints add to the overall financial impact of the disease on society.

Specialized Industries

Because the disease is so widespread, developing drugs to treat arthritis is highly profitable for pharmaceutical companies. For example, *Business Week* magazine, examining the record of the pharmaceutical industry in 1998, predicted that just one of several new arthritis drugs being released at that time could generate sales of $900 million in the year 2001.[11]

Arthritis has also spurred many other forms of specialized industry. Because arthritis sufferers find many everyday tasks difficult, individuals and companies have developed specialized devices to aid them. These include everything from enlarged holders that fit over pens, making them easier to hold, to electronic devices that will open letters and lick stamps. There are special types of eating utensils, such as knives with pistol grips, and angled forks and spoons that make eating easier for people with limited wrist or elbow motion. Reachers, or grabbers, which are long rods with open-jaw pincers at one end to grasp an object, are very popular.

Adaptive clothing for people with arthritis may feature Velcro® instead of buttons or zippers, and have roomier armholes for easier sliding on and off. There are also buttoners and unbuttoners, zipper openers, sock and shoe aids, and other devices to help people with arthritis get dressed.

For the bathroom, arthritis sufferers can buy comb grippers, electric toothbrushes, special squeeze containers for toothpaste, seats for the tub, safety rails, and raised toilet seats. Pill-cap openers can help people with crippled hands open their pill bottles.

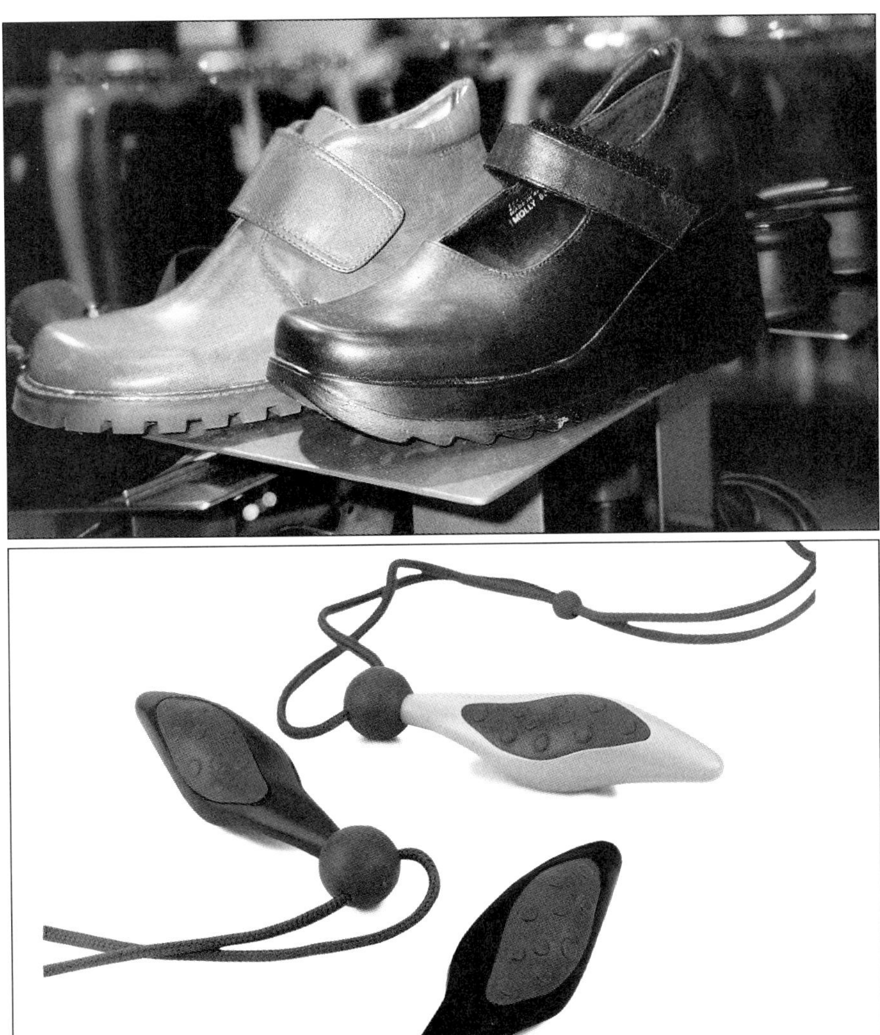

Many manufacturers make specially designed products that can help a person with arthritis perform daily tasks (although many people without arthritis buy these products, too). Here are shoes with Velcro® straps and easy-to-grip pens.

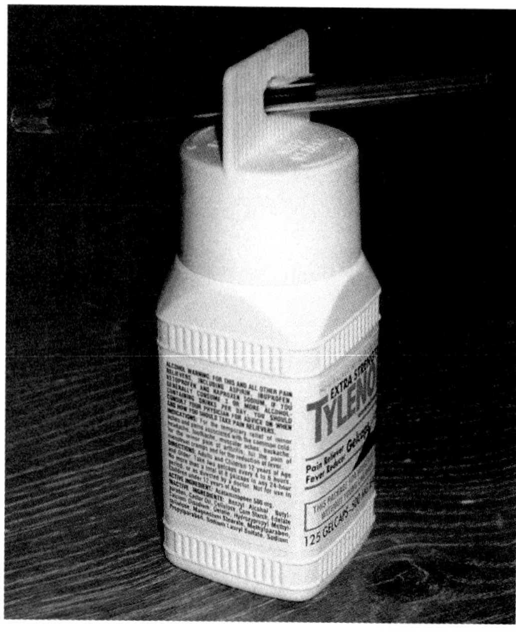

By inserting an ordinary pen or pencil through the special cap on this medicine bottle, a person with arthritis can open the bottle easily.

In addition, of course, there are factories turning out canes, crutches, walkers, wheelchairs, and three-wheeled power chairs.

Despite the manufacture and sale of all these drugs and devices, their boost to the economy is easily outweighed by the cost of treating arthritis. This disease remains an enormous problem for society at the individual, family, national, and international levels.

7

Preventing Arthritis

Boomer Esiason, former quarterback for the Cincinnati Bengals, the New York Jets, and the St. Louis Cardinals, once thought his football career was over, almost before it began.

"When I was fourteen years old, I started having extreme pain," he says. "The doctor diagnosed arthritis and prescribed twenty-four aspirin a day. I'll never forget how badly it hurt when they drained my knee. But the pain was minor compared to the fear.

"You see, I was just going into ninth grade and all I wanted to do was to play football. But all this happened in June, and football started in August."

Fortunately for Esiason—and for the Cincinnati Bengals—his childhood disease went into remission and has not returned. However, Esiason also knows that a different type of arthritis may someday figure in his future. "Among retired football players, osteoarthritis is the number one ailment," he says. "After punishing my body with the on-the-field licks and bruises all these years, I know my chances of developing arthritis later in life are greater than average."[1]

Esiason's experience shows how difficult it is to prevent arthritis. There was nothing he could do to prevent his juvenile rheumatoid arthritis. As for osteoarthritis, although its onset may be postponed by avoiding activities that put excessive wear and tear on the joints, that is not always a practical course of action. It is doubtful that Esiason would have given up the chance to lead the Cincinnati Bengals to the 1988 Super Bowl, even if it might have put off the development of osteoarthritis sometime down the road!

Risk Factors

In order to try to prevent or at least postpone the onset of arthritis, you first have to know who is most likely to get it. That was the focus of a report released in 1996 by the Centers for Disease Control in Atlanta, Georgia. The report compared many previous studies to determine which of a number of unrelated risk factors were most important. It found that advancing age and overweight were the conditions that put people at the highest risk for arthritis. As we saw earlier, women are also more likely to get arthritis than men.

In addition, there is increasing evidence that at least some of the risk of developing arthritis is inherited. Doctors have known for a long time that arthritis sometimes clusters in families. However, only recently have researchers begun to zero in on the specific genes that pass the predisposition for arthritis from generation to generation.[2] Much more research in this field remains to be done.

At the other end of the scale, the single most important factor in determining the risk of arthritis was race: Asians, Pacific islanders, and Hispanics had the lowest risk of arthritis. A higher education level was also associated with a lower risk of arthritis.[3]

Most of these risk factors are out of our control. We can't pick our ancestors. You're either born Asian or Hispanic, or you're not. There's not much you can do about whether you're male or female, either. And no matter how hard we try not to, we all get older.

However, one factor is at least partially within our control: weight.

The reason heavier people tend to suffer more from arthritis is simple: extra weight puts more strain on the joints. Every pound of body weight increases the forces to which your knees are subjected by six pounds, and increases the forces on your hips by three pounds.[4] In other words, says Toronto nutritionist Dr. John Lefebvre, "If you put on ten pounds of extra weight, you're carrying an extra sixty pounds across your knees every time you walk. Twenty pounds isn't a lot of weight, but that translates into 120 pounds of force every time you take a step." That means a little extra weight can add up to a lot of wear and tear. An ongoing long-term study, which began in

1948, involving much of the adult population of Framingham, Massachusetts, has shown that weight loss over a ten-year period cut in half the risk of osteoarthritis in the knees of overweight women middle-aged and older.[5]

It does not take an enormous weight loss to make a difference, either. Reducing one's weight by just ten pounds decreases the risk of developing osteoarthritis by 50 percent. It also helps those who have already developed the disease. "A study showed that if people [with osteoarthritis] lost weight, the amount of pain and discomfort they experienced decreased dramatically," says Lefebvre.[6]

Although keeping weight down and avoiding joint injuries may reduce the risk of osteoarthritis, most forms of arthritis have no known method of prevention. That is because we do not yet know what causes them.

There are a few exceptions. Prompt treatment of Lyme disease with antibiotics, for instance, can keep the form of arthritis it causes from appearing. Gout sufferers can help avoid attacks by drinking less alcohol and avoiding fatty meats.

For most arthritis patients, however, their hope is limited to preventing some of the pain and suffering their disease might otherwise cause.

Coping with Arthritis

Besides drugs and surgery, other methods are available to help patients control their disease and keep it from completely taking over their lives.

Preventing Lyme Disease

Lyme Disease is caused by an infection passed from deer to humans by a tick. Here are some simple precautions you can take to avoid being infected:

- Use insect repellent that contains deet when going into wooded areas;
- Wear protective clothing, such as long-sleeved shirts and long pants tucked into high socks;
- Check your clothing and your entire body carefully for ticks;
- Remove any ticks you find carefully using tweezers—make sure you remove both the head and the body;
- Make sure your dogs or cats wear flea and tick collars and are treated with tick-preventive medications, since pets can carry the ticks into your home.

If you are bitten, you may not even be aware of it. If you develop any fever, headache, or other flu-like symptoms, examine your body carefully for a circular rash with a bright red outer border. Although not everyone infected with Lyme disease develops it, this characteristic rash does indicate you have been infected. Blood tests are available to confirm your suspicions. Treatment of the infection with antibiotics at this early stage can prevent more serious symptoms later, including arthritis.

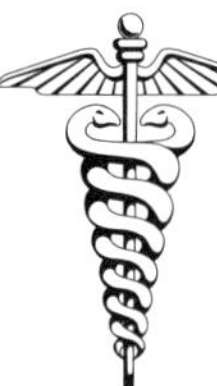

Recommendations for Preventing or Reducing the Effects of Arthritis[7]

Seek early diagnosis and treatment. It is important to find out if you have arthritis and what type it is because treatments vary for each type. Early diagnosis and treatment are important to help slow or prevent damage to joints that can occur during the first few years. If consulting a family doctor, discuss the need for timely referral to specialty care.

Maintain appropriate weight. Maintaining your appropriate weight, especially for women, can reduce the risks for developing osteoarthritis in the knees, and possibly in the hips and hands. Research shows that middle-aged and older women of average height who lose eleven pounds or more over ten years cut their risk for developing osteoarthritis of the knees in half. In men, excessive weight also increases the risk for developing gout.

Protect joints. Joint injuries caused by accidents or overuse increase your risk for osteoarthritis. Keeping the muscles around joints strong—especially the knee—may reduce the risk of wear on that joint.

Exercise. Regular physical activity helps build and maintain healthy bones, muscles, and joints. In addition, studies show that exercise helps reduce pain and fatigue.

Practice self-care strategies. Be a good arthritis manager. Contact your local chapter of the Arthritis Foundation for more information on understanding your disease, knowing what to expect, tips for working with your health-care team, and programs and services available in your area.

One method is exercise. Strong muscles are better able to support and protect joints. "Several studies show that if you improve muscle strength, you decrease pain," says Dennis Boulware, a rheumatologist at the University of Alabama in Birmingham. Although joints will probably hurt during the exercise, they should not still be hurting so intensely several hours later.[8]

If they do, the patient has probably done too much. "There's a fine line between doing too much and too little," says William Ginsburg, a rheumatologist at the Mayo Clinic in Jacksonville, Florida. "Sometimes people have to be reminded to slow down and listen to their disease."[9]

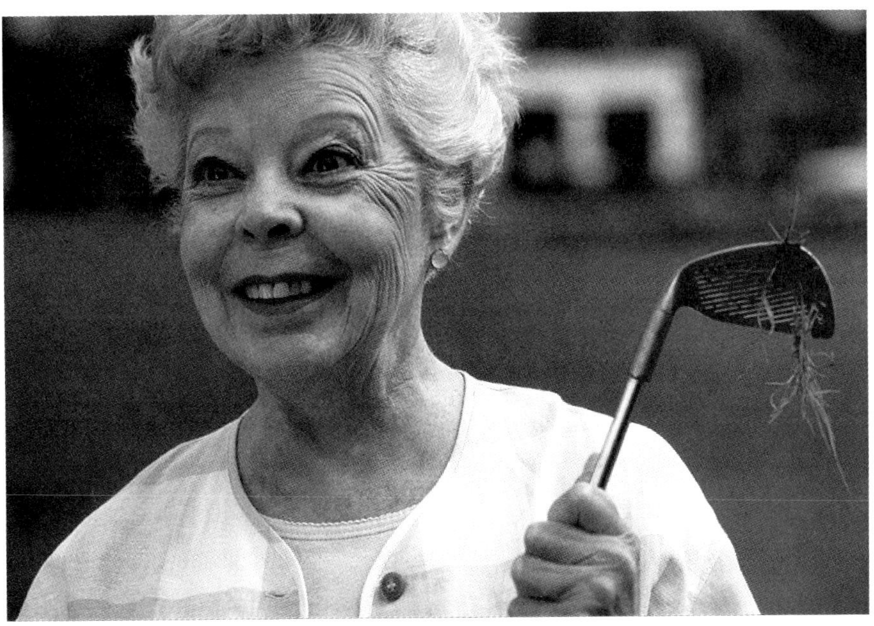

Exercise is one important method to control the advance of arthritis. Strong muscles are better able to support and protect the joints.

That's another way of saying that whereas exercise is important in keeping arthritis from becoming crippling, so is rest. Arthritis patients are urged to take short breaks and alternate heavy and light activities during the day so they don't place too much stress on their joints or get too tired. The balance between rest and exercise must be flexible as the disease flares up or quiets down. Arthritis communicates to those suffering from it through pain. If pain increases during or after an activity or exercise, then the person is probably doing too much. If it lasts more than two hours after a task is completed, that's a sign the person should not try to perform that same task in the same way next time.

Reducing stress on the joints can be done through a number of methods, most of which are based on good body mechanics—using all the parts of the body wisely.

One basic element of reducing stress on the joints is to practice good posture—whether standing, sitting, or lying down. Another method is to distribute weighty loads over the stronger joints and larger surface areas. An example of this strategy would be to carry a purse on the shoulder instead of in the hand.

Joint stress can also be reduced by lifting objects when they are close to the body instead of with the arms extended. Another important tip is to move or change position often. This movement keeps joints from stiffening up. People who suffer from rheumatoid arthritis are particularly susceptible to having joints stiffen if they are not moved regularly. This stiffening process is called "gelling."[10]

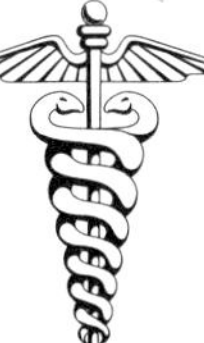

Body Mechanics Tips for People With Arthritis

Arthritis makes people struggle with simple actions the rest of us take for granted—like getting up from a chair. These tips, taken from the Arthritis Foundation's brochure *Managing Your Activities,* will give you some idea of how arthritis can affect everyday activities.

- When lifting something that is low or on the ground, bend your knees and lift by straightening your legs.
- Use reachers—poles with a jaw at one end and a grip to open and close the jaw at the other—instead of bending to pick up something from the floor or reaching above in high cupboards.
- If you have to bend, try to keep your back straight and bend using your knees.
- To get up from a chair, slide forward to the edge. Keep your feet flat on the floor. Lean forward, then push down with your palms—not your fingers—on the arms or seat of the chair. If you have wrist pain, you can push off using your forearms against the top of your thighs. Stand up by straightening your hips and knees.

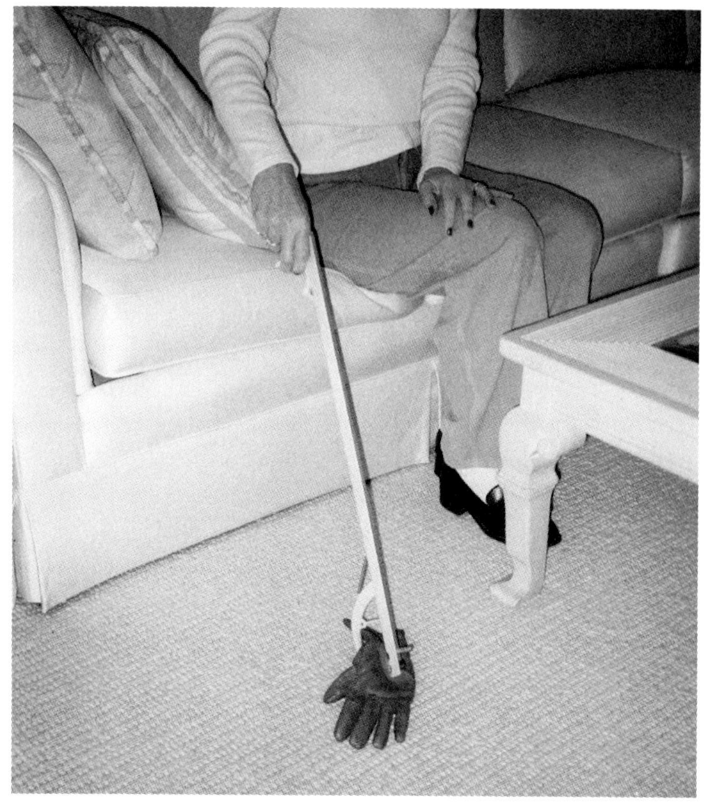

Picking up objects with specially designed reachers can help people who are not able to bend easily.

Another way to reduce stress on the joints is to make use of widely available mechanical devices. These range from simple, everyday devices like an electric knife for cutting roasts (much easier to use than a regular carving knife for someone with arthritis in their hands) and an electric can-opener to devices more specifically designed for people with arthritis, such as raised toilet seats and grab bars in the bathroom and, in more severe cases, canes and walkers.

8

Research and the Future

Rheumatology, the study of arthritis, is one of the most active fields of research in medicine. Since the 1940s doctors have learned how to classify, diagnose, and manage many forms of arthritis, such as chronic gout, lupus, and arthritis associated with rheumatic fever. Still, a lot remains to be done, and research is continuing.

Research into arthritis can be broken down into two broad categories: research into new treatments, and research into the disease process and its causes. In general, research into why and how arthritis begins points the way to the new treatments.

Searching for the Cause

One focus of current research is on the immune system. There are hundreds of research teams working on various aspects of the immune system. Many of these research teams are not focusing on arthritis specifically, but every bit of knowledge gained helps other scientists who are working on arthritis.

Many researchers are studying abnormalities in the immune systems of people with rheumatoid arthritis and in animals with a similar disease. Understanding these abnormalities could lead to ways to stop inflammation very early, before it causes serious damage.

A few years ago scientists in Canada, England, the United States, and Italy discovered that rheumatoid arthritis could be triggered by an "infectious agent"—in other words, a germ. A bacteria found in most people's intestines, called *Escherichia coli*, or *E. coli*, is one possible culprit.[1] If a germ helps trigger rheumatoid arthritis, some scientists believe, it might be possible to develop an arthritis vaccine.

Some scientists are exploring the possibility that arthritis might be triggered by some kind of germ that is able to disguise itself so that it looks very much like something that normally occurs in the body. This "molecular mimicry" could fool the body into creating antibodies that attack its own tissues.[2]

Looking at Genetics

Another major focus of current research into the causes of arthritis is genetics. One major study currently underway is called the North American Rheumatoid Arthritis Consortium. Twelve research centers around the United States are collecting information and genetic material from a thousand families in which two or more siblings have rheumatoid arthritis. The data collected will help other researchers track down any hereditary component of the disease.[3]

In another project, scientists are studying rats with a form of arthritis similar to rheumatoid arthritis in humans. They have already found several components of the rats' genes that are related to how likely they are to get arthritis. This discovery could help us find the same types of genetic material in human genes.[4] However, it is a difficult process, because it seems likely that many different genes play a role in the development of arthritis.

One recent success in genetic research has been the discovery of a gene that may be linked to the faulty development of cartilage, which in turn could lead to the development of osteoarthritis.

Other bodily processes that may contribute to the development of arthritis are also under study. For example, scientists are studying the structure of cartilage and the cells that keep it healthy. Scientists want to know why, in osteoarthritis, the cartilage breaks down faster than it can be repaired.

In addition, they are examining how bones move and fit together at the joints, and how joints react to various stresses and strains. This may not only give us a better understanding of how joint damage can lead to osteoarthritis, it may also show us how we can avoid further damage.

The influence of hormones on arthritis is also under study. Some scientists are trying to find out whether the normal changes in the levels of hormones, such as estrogen and testosterone, during a lifetime are related to the development of the disease or its course. These studies are also aimed at finding out why so many more women than men develop arthritis.

It now appears likely that there is not one single cause of most forms of arthritis. Instead, the disease probably arises through the complex interaction of many different factors. For example, a person with a certain genetic makeup, who is infected by a certain virus at a certain time in life, might get arthritis, whereas someone else with the same genetic makeup who avoided infection might not.

Because there are so many factors involved, it doesn't seem likely that a single treatment will work for everyone, either. However, new treatments are being developed all the time.

Seeking Better Treatments

One of the main focuses of research into arthritis treatments is to find anti-inflammatory drugs with fewer side effects than those available now. The Cox-2 inhibitors are one example.

Currently many researchers are experimenting with new drugs called "biopharmaceuticals" or "biologics." These are drugs that are based on compounds that occur naturally in the body, and are designed to attack the excessive number of white blood cells in an inflamed joint.[5]

"Some biologics are incredibly powerful," says Dr. Ed Keystone, director of the rheumatic disease unit at Toronto's Wellesley Hospital. "After a single injection, an RA [rheumatoid arthritis] patient may go into remission for months, even a year. Studies show that some patients do very well after a single infusion of these agents and need no other therapy."[6]

Now severe cases of rheumatoid arthritis are sometimes treated with drugs that have, as one of their side effects, the result of reducing the effectiveness of the immune system. Unfortunately, these drugs wipe out the cells the body needs to fight off infections like colds. Biologics are more like guided missiles; they are designed to attack specific cells, preserving those cells the body needs to fight infections. Keystone thinks biologics, in combination with other medications, may eventually be able to help as many as one quarter of rheumatoid arthritis patients.[7]

Another experimental way to treat the kinds of arthritis in which the immune system attacks the body is to create custom antibodies. These special antibodies attack the cells that start the misguided immune response or some of the proteins in the blood that promote inflammation.

One of those proteins is called tumor necrosis factor, or TNF. Large amounts of TNF can be found in the fluid surrounding arthritis-infected joints. When it is present, the body creates white blood cells that cause the cells lining the joint to become sticky and sop up even more white blood cells. "When things get really nasty, it [TNF] actually chews away at the bone, eroding it," explains Dr. David Fox, chief of rheumatology at the University of Michigan in Ann Arbor. One new class of drugs, called tumor necrosis factor antagonists, soaks up excess TNF before it can cause joint damage. Combining this type of drug with another arthritis medication, methotrexate, works better than methotrexate alone, according to a recent study.[8]

A New Treatment for Juvenile Arthritis

In February 1999, results from another new study pointed the way to a possible new treatment for severe juvenile arthritis. In the study, four children, aged six to eleven, received bone marrow transplants after standard drug treatments failed to halt their arthritis.

Dr. Nico Wulffraat and colleagues from Utrecht, the Netherlands, first collected marrow from the bones in the children's hips. Bone marrow contains immature cells called stem cells that can form all the different cells of the blood system. The doctors treated the bone marrow cells with antibodies designed to fight the white blood cells causing the inflammation, then injected the treated cells back into the children's bodies.

After six to eighteen months, joint swelling had gone down in all the children. The children were not in nearly as much pain, and they no longer needed to take other drugs. The researchers are still watching these children to see if any symptoms of their disease return.[9]

The wide variety of research being carried out into the causes of arthritis and the many different types of treatment being tried reflect the complexity of the disease. That complexity makes it unlikely that a full cure will be found any time soon. But recent advances offer the hope that within a few more years, far fewer people will be suffering from arthritis the way they are suffering now.

With arthritis, reducing suffering is always a doctor's first and most important goal.

Q & A

Q. What is arthritis?

A. Arthritis is an inflammation of the joints. It can be caused by more than one hundred different conditions. Its severity can range from a mild annoyance to a completely crippling disability.

Q. I've heard of people having hips or knees replaced. When do doctors use surgery to treat arthritis?

A. Surgery is considered when arthritis doesn't respond well to other treatments and the patient is in constant pain. Replacing a joint can relieve pain and increase mobility. However, artificial joints don't last forever and may have to be replaced.

Q. How do I know if I have arthritis?

A. If you have pain, stiffness, or swelling in or around a joint for more than two weeks, it's time to see your doctor. Only a doctor can tell if you have arthritis.

Q. My grandmother moved to Arizona because she said the warm weather would help her arthritis. Does that really work?

A. Some people feel better in a warm, dry climate. Studies have shown that rheumatoid arthritis symptoms get worse when the barometric pressure goes down and humidity goes up—when it's going to rain, for example. However, a warmer, drier climate does not cure the disease.

Q. What are the best medications for arthritis?

A. Arthritis is a different disease for everyone who has it, so no one medication works equally well on everyone. With osteoarthritis, pain may be the main problem, so the doctor may prescribe a painkiller. With rheumatoid arthritis and lupus, where inflammation is the main problem, medications called nonsteroidal anti-inflammatory drugs (NSAIDs) are often prescribed. Aspirin is one of them; others have to be bought with a prescription. Doctors have many more powerful drugs they can try, as well.

Q. Is there any way to keep from getting arthritis?

A. We don't know what causes most forms of arthritis, so there isn't much we can do to prevent them. However, it's a good idea to maintain your recommended weight, avoid joint injuries from overuse or accidents, and exercise regularly.

Q. Can anyone get arthritis?

A. Yes. Various forms of arthritis affect infants to senior citizens. However, different forms of arthritis are more prevalent in different age groups. People over fifty are more likely to get osteoarthritis than young people, for example. In addition, arthritis affects three women for every two men.

Q. Is there a cure for arthritis?

A. There is no known cure for most forms of arthritis. You'll see many "cures" for arthritis advertised in magazines and on the Internet. Patients should check with their doctors before trying any such treatments. They could be wasting their money or even endangering their health.

Q. Does knuckle-cracking cause arthritis?

A. Knuckle-cracking does not cause arthritis or any other kind of joint damage. The cracking sound is caused by changes in pressure in the joint capsule.

Q. My mother has arthritis. Will I get it, too?

A. Susceptibility to some forms of arthritis may be inherited. However, only a small percentage of the people who are susceptible to arthritis actually get it.

Arthritis Timeline[1]

123 A.D.—A text from India called *Caraka Samhita* describes a disease where swollen, painful joints initially appear in the hands and feet, then spread to include other parts of the body, causing loss of appetite and occasionally fever.

1200s—The Dominican monk Randolfus of Bocking, England, describes gout as an episodic swelling of the big toe. He is the first to see it as a separate disease.

1591—Guillaume de Baillou (1538–1616), a French physician and dean of the University of Paris medical faculty, prepares one of the first books to be written on arthritis. He uses the term *rheumatisme* to describe a condition characterized by inflammation, soreness, stiffness in the muscles, and pain in and around the joints.

1670s—Dutchman Anton van Leeuwenhoek uses a simple microscope to identify crystals in the blood or synovial fluid that are characteristic of gout.

1676—Thomas Sydenham, an English physician, writes of a long-term, chronic, debilitating disease that affects many joints and causes deformity in the joints of the fingers. He was probably describing rheumatoid arthritis.

1680s—Peruvian bark, which contains the antimalarial agent quinine, is used to treat rheumatic disorders. Medical records from this time indicate that physical exercise is advocated for chronic arthritis.

1763—English clergyman Edmund Stone notes that willow bark remedies (which contain salicylate, the active ingredient that will later be used to make aspirin) help reduce rheumatic fever and pain.

1816—Sir Charles Scudmore of England notes that arthritis runs in families.

1820—Salicylate is isolated from natural sources by Italian, German, and French scientists.

1850—French neurologist Guillaume Benjamin Arman Duchenne (1806–1875) describes several arthritic and muscular disorders for the first time.

1854—Sir Alfred Garrod, a London physician, devises tests to detect uric acid in the blood and urine of gout sufferers. He correctly hypothesizes that gout results either from the kidneys being unable to process uric acid properly, or from a buildup of uric acid in the system.

1855—Remains of a Neanderthal man unearthed in Germany show signs of arthritis, proving the disease dates back at least one hundred fifty thousand years.

1859—London physician Sir Alfred Garrod coins the clinical term *rheumatoid arthritis.*

1863—English surgeon John Hilton publishes *Rest and Pain*, which recommends periods of rest to help manage arthritis.

1872—In one of the earliest identifications of systemic lupus erythematosus, Vienna's Moriz Kaposi uses the term *disseminated lupus erythematosus* to describe disorders where there are widespread skin lesions, fever, chest inflammation, and joint inflammation and pain.

1888—John Kent Spender, a physician in Bath, England, names osteoarthritis.

1890—At the nineteenth Congress of the German Society for Surgery, surgeons outline the general concepts for total joint replacement. Current joint replacement methods are still based on these concepts.

1893—The surgeon W. A. Lane develops a system of carbon steel screws and plates that makes internal repair of bones and joints possible.

1895—Wilhelm Roentgen, a German scientist, identifies X rays, which become an essential tool for diagnosing joint and bone problems.

1897—The Bayer Company in Germany synthesizes a new pain reliever, acetylsalicylic acid, better known as aspirin. It quickly gains worldwide recognition in the treatment of pain and rheumatic disorders.

1907—Swiss physician Fritz Steinman introduces a special pin that makes further progress in joint repair possible.

1908—Sir Grafton Elliot Smith, chair of the anatomy department at the government medical school in Cairo, Egypt, notes evidence of ankylosing spondylitis in skeletons of young men unearthed from Egyptian and Nubian tombs thousands of years old.

1919—After World War I, Sir Robert Jones of Liverpool, England, and other surgeons around the world develop orthopedic surgery as a medical specialty that focuses on preserving and restoring the functions of the skeletal system.

1923—The first public survey to measure the social and economic impact of rheumatoid arthritis is taken in Sweden. This, together with another study in England the following year, first draws public attention to the importance of this field of medicine. The English study shows that a sixth of all human industrial incapacity is caused by rheumatism and arthritis.

1926—Developed fourteen years earlier, stainless steel is used as a corrosion-resistant material for orthopedic implant devices.

1929—Periodic injections of gold salts are first used to relieve arthritis pain.

1930—Sir McFarlane Burnet, head of the Research Institute of Melbourne, Australia, asserts that autoimmunity, the process by which the body's defense system malfunctions and attacks its own tissues, causes many arthritic conditions.

1931—Boston surgeon Marius Smith-Petersen introduces a three-pronged nail that secures the ball joint in hip fixation procedures, and develops a metal cup for use in partial hip replacement.

1933—The American Academy of Orthopaedic Surgeons is formed in Chicago.

1938—Surgeons in England perform the first total hip replacement.

1941—Rheumatoid arthritis is officially recognized as a distinct disorder by the American Rheumatism Association.

1948—The Arthritis Foundation is established. Doctors Philip Hench and E. C. Kendall discover the therapeutic anti-inflammatory effects of steroid hormones, and later win the Nobel Prize for their discovery.

The rheumatoid factor, an antibody that indicates an important disturbance in a person's immune mechanisms, is isolated in the blood of rheumatoid arthritis sufferers.

1949—The use of corticosteroids transforms systemic lupus erythematosus (lupus), which was almost always fatal, into a manageable disease.

1955—Prednisone, a synthetic derivative of cortisone, is introduced and quickly becomes the most widely used oral corticosteroid medication.

1959—British orthopedic surgeon Sir John Charnley begins extensive research and innovations in low-friction total hip replacement. He revolutionizes modern total hip replacement.

1975—The National Arthritis Act is established to study arthritis; authorize grants; and set up a data bank, an information clearinghouse, and comprehensive centers to promote research, diagnosis, treatment, rehabilitation, and education around musculoskeletal disorders.

A mysterious form of arthritis occurs among people in Lyme, Connecticut, and surrounding towns. Medical researchers soon recognize the illness as a distinct disease, which they name Lyme disease.

1982—Sir John Vane, an English pharmacologist, receives the Nobel Prize in physiology for his discovery of prostaglandins, biological substances that are responsible for the characteristics of inflammation—pain, redness, stiffness, and warmth—and for his explanation of how aspirin counters inflammation.

1990—The Americans with Disabilities Act is passed by the United States Congress, requiring that buildings provide equal access to people with disabilities.

Scientists discover that a gene defect is associated with osteoarthritis.

1999—New anti-inflammatory drugs, called Cox-2 inhibitors, which do not have the unpleasant gastrointestinal side effects of previous drugs, become available.

Glossary

ankylosing spondylitis—A type of arthritis that primarily affects the spine. Tendons and ligaments become inflamed where they attach to the bone. Severe cases sometimes result in the formation of bony bridges between the bones, causing the spine to become rigid.

antibody—A protein produced in the blood or tissues, triggered by the immune system, to destroy any substance considered foreign or threatening to the body.

antigen—Any substance the body recognizes as foreign or a possible threat. Its appearance in the body will stimulate production of an antibody.

arthrodesis—Fusing joint bones together surgically to relieve pain.

arthroplasty—Surgical reconstruction of a joint using the patient's own tissue.

arthroscopy—Examination of the inside of a joint by inserting a slender optical instrument, an endoscope, through a small incision.

autoimmune disease—A disease caused by the malfunctioning of the immune system so that it attacks the body's own tissues.

bacteria—A self-contained microscopic organism that eats, excretes, and reproduces.

bursa—A tiny sac that acts as a cushion between muscles and bones. It releases a fluid that lubricates muscles, tendons, and bones so they can slide smoothly over each other.

bursitis—Inflammation of a bursa.

cartilage—A flexible material that cushions the ends of the bones in a joint so they don't rub together.

chronic—Persisting over a long period of time.

complete blood count (CBC)—A blood test that counts the white blood cells, red blood cells, and platelets in a sample of blood.

connective tissue—Tissues that support and connect other tissues and organs.

corticosteroids—Drugs given to arthritis patients to reduce the inflammation of the joints. They are a synthetic form of cortisol, a hormone produced by the adrenal glands.

CPPD disease—A form of arthritis caused by crystals of a salt called calcium pyrophosphate dihydrate being deposited in the joints. Pseudogout is one example.

degeneration—Deterioration, especially change of a tissue from a higher to a lower form.

flare—A period of time during which arthritis symptoms become worse.

gelling—The stiffening of joints.

genetics—The branch of biology that studies how characteristics are passed down from generation to generation.

gout—A form of arthritis caused by deposits of monosodium urate crystals in the joints.

immune system—The body's many different methods of identifying and destroying invading organisms and substances.

immunology—A branch of medicine that studies how humans fight off disease.

infectious arthritis—Any form of arthritis caused by a virus or bacteria, such as Lyme disease.

inflammation—The body's reaction to injury or infection. It results in redness, heat, swelling, pain, and loss of function.

joint—A structure where two bones come together. Some allow a wide range of motion; others are fixed.

joint capsule—A fibrous capsule that encloses the joint, including the ends of the bones and the cartilage.

juvenile rheumatoid arthritis—The umbrella term for several types of arthritis that occur in children under age sixteen.

ligaments—Thick fibers that are anchored to the bones on both sides of a joint to keep them in alignment.

lupus—*See* systemic lupus erythematosus.

Lyme disease—An infection of the joints caused by bacteria transmitted by a type of tick.

muscles—Specialized tissues that are able to contract. They support the joints and allow them to move.

nonsteroidal anti-inflammatory drugs (NSAIDs)—Drugs that are not steroids that reduce pain and inflammation. Aspirin is one example.

osteoarthritis—A type of arthritis caused by a degeneration of the cartilage in a joint. This makes joints stiff and painful, but not always inflamed.

osteophytes—Small spurs of bone that form at the ends of bones in joints affected by osteoarthritis.

osteotomy—Surgical removal of bone to allow realignment of a joint.

pauciarticular disease—Any form of arthritis, especially juvenile arthritis, that affects only a few joints.

polyarticular disease—Any form of arthritis, especially juvenile arthritis, that affects many joints.

prostaglandins—Body chemicals that play a key role in inflammation.

pseudogout—*See* CPPD disease.

remission—A lessening or ending of the symptoms of a disease. Also, the period during which such a lessening occurs.

rheumatic fever—An illness that usually follows a streptococcal infection and may lead to a form of arthritis.

rheumatism—An old-fashioned term for any condition that causes pain and swelling in the joints and surrounding tissues.

rheumatoid factor—An antibody found in large amounts in the blood of people with rheumatoid arthritis. Finding it can help a doctor diagnose the disease.

rheumatologist—A doctor who specializes in diagnosing and treating arthritis.

risk factor—A condition that increases a person's chance of developing arthritis (or any other disease), such as age, gender, or family history.

synovial fluid—A thick, clear fluid produced by the synovial membrane that lubricates the joint.

synovial membrane—The inside lining of a joint capsule.

systemic lupus erythematosus—An autoimmune disease that can cause inflammation in various body tissues, including the joints, skin, kidneys, heart, lungs, blood vessels, and brain. Often called lupus, for short.

tendonitis—Inflammation of the tendons.

tendons—Strong bands of tissue that connect bones and muscle.

uric acid—A waste product normally found in the blood. Too much of it in the bloodstream can lead to gout.

virus—An organism that is unable to reproduce on its own. Instead, it invades living cells and tricks them into producing hundreds of new viruses, which spill out when the cell dies and bursts.

For More Information

Organizations

American Juvenile Arthritis Association
1314 Spring Street
Atlanta, GA 30309
(404) 872-7100

The American Lupus Society
23751 Madison Street
Torrance, CA 90505
(213) 373-1335

American Physical Therapy Association
1111 North Fairfax Street
Alexandria, VA 22314
(703) 684-2782
Fax: (703) 684-7343

Ankylosing Spondylitis Association
511 North La Cienega
Suite 216
Los Angeles, CA 90048
(800) 777-8189

The Arthritis Foundation
1314 Spring Street
Atlanta, GA 30309
(404) 872-7100

The Arthritis Society
250 Bloor Street East
Suite 901
Toronto, ON M4W 3P2
(416) 967-1414

Fibromyalgia Alliance of America
P. O. Box 21990
Columbus, OH 43221-0990
(614) 457-4222
Fax: (614) 457-2729

Lupus Foundation of America
1300 Piccard Drive, Suite 200
Rockville, MD 20580-4303
(888) 385-8787
Fax: (301) 670-9486

Lyme Disease Foundation
One Financial Plaza, 18th Floor
Hartford, CT 06103
(860) 525-2000
Fax: (860) 525-8425

National Fibromyalgia Research Association
P. O. Box 500
Salem, OR 97302
(800) 574-3468
Fax: (503) 315-7212

National Marfan Association
328 Main Street
Port Washington, NY 11050
(800) 862-7326
Fax: (516) 883-8040

The Paget Foundation
120 Wall Street, Suite 1602
New York, NY 10005
(800) 237-2438
Fax: (212) 509-8492

Scleroderma Foundation
89 Newbury Street, Suite 201
Danvers, MA 01923-1075
(800) 722-4673
Fax: (978) 750-9902

Spondylitis Association of America
P. O. Box 5872
Sherman Oaks, CA 91413
(800) 777-8189
Fax: (818) 981-9826

Internet Resources

About.com
<http://arthritis.about.com/health/arthritis>

American College of Rheumatology
<http://www.rheumatology.org>

American Physical Therapy Association
<http://www.apta.org>

The Arthritis Foundation
<http://www.arthritis.org>

The Canadian Arthritis Society
<http://www.arthritis.ca>

Discovery Health
<http://www.discoveryhealth.com>

Johns Hopkins Health InteliHealth
<http://www.intelihealth.com>

Lupus Foundation of America
<http://www.lupus.org>

Lyme Disease Foundation
<http://www.lyme.org>

National Databook for Rheumatic Diseases
<http://www.fibromyalgia.org>

National Institutes of Health and National Institute of Arthritis and Musculoskeletal and Skin Diseases
<http://www.nih.gov/niams>

National Marfan Foundation
<http://www.marfan.org>

on**health.com**
<http://onhealth.com>

The Paget Foundation
<http://www.paget.org>

Scleroderma Foundation
<http://www.scleroderma.org>

Spondylitis Association of America
<http://www.spondylitis.org>

University of Washington Department of Orthopaedics Bone and Joint Source
<http://www.orthop.washington.edu/bonejoint>

Chapter Notes

Chapter 1. Oh, My Aching Joints!

1. David S. Pisetsky, M.D., Ph.D., with Susan Flamholtz Trien, *The Duke University Medical Center Book of Arthritis* (New York: Fawcett Columbine, 1991), pp.193–194.

2. Ibid., pp. 71–72.

3. Ibid., p. 12.

4. "Arthritis Fact Sheet," The Arthritis Foundation website, <http://www.arthritis.org/resource/fs/arthritis.asp> (September 3, 1999).

5. "Rheumatoid Arthritis Fact Sheet," The Arthritis Foundation website, <http://www.arthritis.org/resource/fs/rheumatoid.asp> (November 26, 1999).

6. "Osteoarthritis Fact Sheet," The Arthritis Foundation website, <http://www.arthritis.org/resource/fs/osteoarthritis.asp> (November 26, 1999).

7. "Study Shows 23 Million Women in U.S. Have Arthritis," *Jet*, May 22, 1995, p. 62.

8. "Gout Fact Sheet," American College of Rheumatology website, <http://www.rheumatology.org/patients/factsheet/gout.html> (September 8, 1999).

9. MSNBC Staff and Wire Reports, "FDA Approves New Arthritis Drug," MSNBC website, December 31, 1998, <http://www.msnbc.com/news/219750.asp> (September 8, 1999).

10. "Arthritis: Not Just a Condition Your Grandmother Gets," Executive Health's *Good Health Report*, October 1997, p. 1.

11. Peter Pompei, "Osteoarthritis: What to Look for, When to Treat It," *Geriatrics*, August 1996, p. 36.

12. Earl J. Brewer, Jr., and Kathy Cochran Angel, *The Arthritis Sourcebook* (Los Angeles: Lowell House, 1993), p. 6.

13. ”Arthritis: Not Just a Condition Your Grandmother Gets,” Executive Health's *Good Health Report*, October 1997, p. 1.

14. “Arthritis Fact Sheet,” The Arthritis Foundation website, <http://www.arthritis.org/resource/fs/arthritis.asp> (September 3, 1999).

15. Carolyn J. Strange, “Coping with Arthritis in Its Many Forms,” *FDA Consumer*, March, 1996, p. 17.

Chapter 2. A History of Arthritis

1. Bruce Bower, “Arthritic Origins in New World?”, *Science News*, April 9, 1988, p. 232.

2. Johns Hopkins Health, “Arthritis Timeline,” InteliHealth website, <http://www.intelihealth.com> (September 1, 1999).

3. Ibid.

4. Derrick Brewerton, *All About Arthritis: Past, Present, Future* (Cambridge, Mass.: Harvard University Press, 1992), p. 43.

5. Ibid.

6. Johns Hopkins Health, “Arthritis Timeline.”

7. “Gout: The most painful kind of arthritis,” HealthBeat website, March 2, 1999, <http://healthlinks.washington.edu/your_health/hbeat/hb990302.html> (September 8, 1999).

8. Carol Eustice, “Gout: Yesterday and Today,” About.com website, <http://arthritis.tqn.com/library/weekly/aa101498.htm> (September 8, 1999).

9. Carol Eustice, “Did You Know?”, About.com website, <http://arthritis.about.com/library/weekly/aa102897.htm> (September 7, 1999).

10. Johns Hopkins Health, “Arthritis Timeline.”

11. Ibid.

12. Brewerton, p. 98.

13. Johns Hopkins Health, “Arthritis Timeline.”

14. Edward Willett, “Aspirin,” *Regina Leader Post*, September 28, 1996, p. D3.

15. Brewerton, pp. 77–78.

16. Ibid., pp. 79–80.

17. Ibid., p. 125.

18. Johns Hopkins Health, "Arthritis Timeline."

19. "Hench, Philip Showalter," *Microsoft Encarta Encyclopedia*, 1998 edition.

20. Johns Hopkins Health, "Arthritis Timeline."

21. Arthritis Foundation History, The Arthritis Foundation website, <http://www.arthritis.org/about/afhistory.asp> (September 7, 1999).

22. Ibid.

23. "Renior, Pierre-Auguste," Microsoft Encarta Encyclopedia, 1998 edition.

24. "Heilmann, Harry," *Microsoft Encarta Encylopedia*, 1998 edition.

25. Cindy T. McDaniel, "Mickey Mantle: playing hardball against arthritis," *Arthritis Today*, May–June 1989, p. 41.

26. Tim Kurkjian, "Waiting for his chance: Pitcher Britt Burns, in lockout limbo like so many other ballplayers, has had his comeback curtailed," *Sports Illustrated*, March 12, 1990, p. 26.

27. Carol Eustice, "Lucille Ball: Comedienne and Arthritis Sufferer," About.com website, <http://arthritis.about.com/library/weekly/aa072997.htm> (September 8, 1999).

28. Ann Oldenburg, "Coburn Beats Back Tough Disease," *USA Today*, December 29, 1998, p. 2D.

Chapter 3. What Is Arthritis?

1. David S. Pisetsky, M.D., Ph.D., with Susan Flamholtz Trien, *The Duke University Medical Center Book of Arthritis* (New York, Fawcett Columbine, 1991), p. 17.

2. Margaret Gore, *The Arthritis Book* (St. Leonards, NSW, Australia: Allan and Unwin, 1997), pp. 2–3.

3. Ibid., p. 1.

4. Derrick Brewerton, *All About Arthritis: Past, Present, Future* (Cambridge, Mass.: Harvard University Press, 1992), p. 125.

5. Ibid., p. 126.

6. Gore, p. 12.

7. "Arthritis," Encarta Online Deluxe website, <http://encarta.msn.com> (September 8, 1999).

8. Pisetsky and Trien, p. 207.

9. "Juvenile Arthritis Fact Sheet," American College of Rheumatology website, <http://www.rheumatology.org/patients/factsheet/jra.html> (September 8, 1999).

10. Ibid.

11. Gore, p. 29.

12. Pisetsky and Trien, pp. 133–136.

13. Ibid., p. 145.

14. "Systemic Lupus Erythematosus Fact Sheet," American College of Rheumatology website, <http://www.rheumatology.org/patients/factsheet/sle.html> (September 8, 1999).

15. Ibid.

16. Pisetsky and Trien, p. 173.

17. Ibid., pp. 191–192.

18. "Questions and Answers," The Arthritis Foundation website, <http://www.arthritis.org/resource/quick_answers.asp> (September 2, 1999).

Chapter 4. Diagnosing Arthritis

1. Dan Hawaleshka, "Arthritis Attack: New Research Points to Effective Treatments," *Maclean's*, July 15, 1996, p. 44.

2. David S. Pisetsky, M.D., Ph.D., with Susan Flamholtz Trien, *The Duke University Medical Center Book of Arthritis* (New York: Fawcett Columbine, 1991), p. 37.

3. Ibid., p. 41.

4. Ibid., p. 42.

5. Ibid., pp. 41–42.

6. Frederick Matsen III, M.D., ed., "Lab Tests in Arthritis," University of Washington Bone and Joint Center website, <http://www.orthop.washington.edu/bonejoint/xzzzzzlz1_2.html> (September 2, 1999).

7. Pisetsky and Trien, p. 44.

8. Matsen.

9. Pisetsky and Trien, pp. 45–46.

10. Ibid., p. 46.

Chapter 5. Treatment of Arthritis

1. Margaret Gore, *The Arthritis Book* (St. Leonards, NSW, Australia: Allan and Unwin, 1997), pp. 32–33.

2. "Handout on Health: Rheumatoid Arthritis," National Institutes of Health and National Institute of Arthritis and Musculoskeletal and Skin Diseases website, <http://www.nih.gov/niams/healthinfo/rahandout/rahandout_breaks.html> (September 2, 1999).

3. Carolyn J. Strange, "Coping with Arthritis in Its Many Forms," *FDA Consumer*, March 1996, p. 17.

4. David S. Pisetsky, M.D., Ph.D., with Susan Flamholtz Trien, *The Duke University Medical Center Book of Arthritis* (New York: Fawcett Columbine, 1991), p. 237.

5. Strange, p. 17.

6. Pisetsky and Trien, p. 239.

7. MSNBC Staff and Wire Reports, "FDA Approves New Arthritis Drug," MSNBC website, December 31, 1998, <http://www.msnbc.com/news/219750.asp> (September 8, 1999).

8. Arthritis Canada, "The Arthritis Society Welcomes a New and Safer Choice for Canadians Living with Arthritis," Arthritis Canada website, <http://www.arthritis.ca/frames/news.html> (July 15, 1999).

9. Pisetsky and Trien, p. 259.

10. Ibid., pp. 258–261.

11. Ibid., p. 251.

12. Ibid., p. 253.

13. Ibid., p. 254.

14. Ibid., pp. 251–254.

15. Félix Fernández-Madrid, M.D., Ph.D., *Treating Arthritis: Medicine, Myth, and Magic* (New York: Insight Books, 1989), p. 169.

16. Gore, p. 52.

17. "Handout on Health: Rheumatoid Arthritis." <http://www.nih.gov/niams/healthinfo/rahandout/rahandout_breaks.html> (September 2, 1999).

18. Ibid.

19. Ibid.

20. Gore, pp. 54–55.

21. Fernández-Madrid, pp. 108–109.

22. Dr. James Dillard, "She's Drawn to Magnets, but Do They Work?" Alternative Health Column, July 16, 1999, OnHealth website, <http://onhealth.com/ch1/columnist/item,45153.asp> (September 8, 1999).

23. Roderick Jamer, *Living With Arthritis* (Vancouver: Whitecap Books, 1996), p. 193.

24. Ibid., pp. 193–194.

25. Fernández-Madrid, pp. 77–78.

26. Ibid., p. 195.

27. Jamer, pp. 192–193.

28. Norman Brown, "New Hope, Better Treatment for Arthritis Sufferers," *Better Homes and Gardens*, April 1992, p. 56.

Chapter 6. Arthritis and Society

1. Dan Hawaleshka, "Arthritis Attack: New Research Points to Effective Treatments," *Maclean's*, July 15, 1996, p. 45.

2. Carolyn J. Strange, "Coping with Arthritis in Its Many Forms," *FDA Consumer*, March, 1996, p. 17.

3. Norman Brown, "New Hope, Better Treatment for Arthritis Sufferers," *Better Homes and Gardens*, April 1992, p. 56.

4. "Arthritis Fact Sheet," The Arthritis Foundation website, <http://www.arthritis.org/resource/fs/arthritis.asp> (September 3, 1999).

5. Roderick Jamer, *Living With Arthritis* (Vancouver: Whitecap Books, 1996), p. 3.

6. "Osteoarthritis Fact Sheet," American College of Rheumatology website, <http://www.rheumatology.org/patients/factsheet/oa.html>.

7. Johns Hopkins Health, "Arthritis Timeline," InteliHealth website, <http://www.intelihealth.com> (September 1, 1999).

8. "Treating Wear and Tear of Joints," *USA Today*, February, 1996.

9. "Rheumatoid Arthritis Fact Sheet," American College of Rheumatology website, <http://www.rheumatology.org/patients/factsheet/ra.html> (September 8, 1999).

10. "What is the Financial Cost of Arthritis?", *The Globe and Mail*, September 1, 1999, p. C2.

11. "Osteoarthritis Fact Sheet."

Chapter 7. Preventing Arthritis

1. Cindy T. McDaniel, "Boomer Esiason: Scoring Against Arthritis," *Arthritis Today*, September–October 1998, p. 27.

2. Centers for Disease Control, "Factors Associated with Prevalent Self-Reported Arthritis and Other Rheumatic Conditions—United States, 1989–1991," *Morbidity and Mortality Weekly Report 45(23)*, June 14, 1996, pp. 487–491.

3. Roderick Jamer, *Living With Arthritis* (Vancouver: Whitecap Books, 1996), p. 185.

4. Tim Lougheed, "Weighing Up the Evidence: A New Study Proves Shedding Pounds Reduces Risk of OA," *Arthritis News*, 1993, The Arthritis Society website, <http://www.arthritis.ca/articles/93r1.html> (November 30, 1999).

5. Jamer, p. 185.

6. David S. Pisetsky, M.D., Ph.D., with Susan Flamholtz Trien, *The Duke University Medical Center Book of Arthritis* (New York: Fawcett Columbine, 1991), pp. 175–176.

7. "The Arthritis Foundation's Recommendations for Preventing or Reducing the Effects of Arthritis," The Arthritis Foundation website, <http://www.arthritis.org/resource/fs/reduce_effects.asp> (September 8, 1999).

8. Carolyn J. Strange, "Coping With Arthritis in Its Many Forms," *FDA Consumer*, March, 1996, p. 17.

9. Ibid.

10. Earl J. Brewer, Jr., M.D., and Kathy Cochran Angel, *The Arthritis Sourcebook* (Los Angeles: Lowell House, 1993), p. 7.

Chapter 8. Research and the Future

1. "Questions and Answers About Arthritis and Rheumatic Disease," National Institute of Arthritis and Musculoskeletal and Skin Diseases website, <http://www.nih.gov/niams/healthinfo/artrheu.htm> (September 8, 1999).

2. David S. Pisetsky, M.D., Ph.D., with Susan Flamholtz Trien, *The Duke University Medical Center Book of Arthritis* (New York: Fawcett Columbine, 1991), p. 368.

3. Ibid.

4. Ibid.

5. Roderick Jamer, *Living With Arthritis* (Vancouver: Whitecap Books, 1996), p. 262.

6. Ibid.

7. Ibid.

8. "Designer Drug Combo Fights Arthritis," MSNBC website, <http://www.msnbc.com/news/210972.asp> (September 8, 1999).

9. "Marrow Transplant May Help Treat Juvenile Rheumatoid Arthritis," Doctor's Guide website, <http://www.pslgroup.com/dg/e50e2.htm> (September 8, 1999).

Timeline

1. Johns Hopkins Health, "Arthritis Timeline," InteliHealth website, <http://www.intelihealth.com> (September 8, 1999).

Further Reading

Aldape, Virginia Tortorica, with Lillian S. Kossacoff (photographer). *Nicole's Story: A Book About a Girl With Juvenile Rheumatoid Arthritis.* Minneapolis, Minn.: Lerner Publications Company, 1996.

Brewer, Earl J. Jr., M.D., and Kathy Cochran Angel. *The Arthritis Sourcebook.* Los Angeles, Calif.: Lowell House, 1993.

Brewerton, Derrick. *All About Arthritis: Past, Present, Future.* Cambridge, Mass.: Harvard University Press, 1992.

Gold, Susan Dudley, and Brian J. Keroack. *Arthritis.* Parsippany, N.J.: Crestwood House, 1997.

Gore, Margaret. *The Arthritis Book.* St. Leonards, NSW, Australia: Allan and Unwin, 1997.

Jamer, Roderick. *Living With Arthritis.* Vancouver: Whitecap Books, 1996.

Pisetsky, David S., M.D., Ph.D., with Susan Flamholtz Trien. *The Duke University Medical Center Book of Arthritis.* New York: Fawcett Columbine, 1991.

Shenkman, Dr. John. *Living With Arthritis* (Living With series). Danbury, Conn.: Franklin Watts, Inc., 1990.

Index